THE WELLNESS REVELATION

THE
WELLNESS
REVELATION

LOSE WHAT WEIGHS YOU DOWN SO YOU CAN
LOVE GOD, YOURSELF, AND OTHERS

FOUNDER OF REVELATION WELLNESS
ALISA KEETON

TYNDALE
MOMENTUM™

*The nonfiction imprint of
Tyndale House Publishers, Inc.*

Visit Tyndale online at www.tyndale.com.

Visit Tyndale Momentum online at www.tyndalemomentum.com.

Visit Alisa Keeton at www.revelationwellness.org.

TYNDALE, *Tyndale Momentum*, and Tyndale's quill logo are registered trademarks of Tyndale House Publishers, Inc. The Tyndale Momentum logo is a trademark of Tyndale House Publishers, Inc. Tyndale Momentum is the nonfiction imprint of Tyndale House Publishers, Inc., Carol Stream, Illinois.

The Wellness Revelation: Lose What Weighs You Down So You Can Love God, Yourself, and Others

Designed by Ron Kaufmann

The stories in this book are about real people and real events, but some names have been changed and some details omitted to protect the privacy of the people involved.

For information about special discounts for bulk purchases, please contact Tyndale House Publishers at csresponse@tyndale.com, or call 1-800-323-9400.

ISBN 978-1-4964-2247-7

Printed in the United States of America

23   22   21   20   19   18   17
7   6   5   4   3   2   1

For my warrior husband, Simon, and my two sharp arrows, Jack and Sophia; your love never quits. You see all my messy parts, and still you call me yours. To receive your love and give you love is God's greatest gift (and training tool) to me. Together we will see the goodness of the Lord in the land of the living.

CONTENTS

Note from the Author

The Wellness Revelation is designed to start you on a journey toward health and wholeness, but it is not intended as a substitute for medical advice from your health care professionals. Revelation Wellness is neither a nutritional consultancy nor a medical provider. Before making significant changes to your diet and exercise routines, it's important that you consult with your own physician.

INTRODUCTION

As a fitness instructor for more than two decades, I've seen the same two clients over and over again. Initially, it was difficult to tell them apart.

The first one enthusiastically embraced all the cardio sweating, the muscle training, and the recommended "do and do not" food lists. Her face lit up as she described the half marathon she was training for. But then something changed: That enthusiasm turned into obsession, and she became less delighted and more driven as she sought to push her BMI just a little lower and the number of dumbbell curls just a little higher. She no longer exuded joy but instead an anxious intensity. At some point, I longed to tell this client, "I can't offer you any other ideas on how to obtain the perfect body if you keep moving the target on me."

The second client also dove right into the workouts, and she sounded pleased when she told me about the weekend she spent purging her pantry of all products with refined flour and added sweeteners. She, too, was delighted to see her body responding to her efforts. But then something happened. Maybe her toddler came down with a nasty bug, or her work schedule changed. She began missing her early morning workouts and canceled her meetings with our nutritionist. Then one day I realized I hadn't seen her in a couple of weeks, so I called and left a message telling her that I missed seeing her. I was so happy when I spotted her at the grocery store—but I stopped myself from saying hello after she turned red when she saw me and ducked down the bread aisle. The smell of shame filled the air. I wanted to tell her, "I still see and value you. You were never just a body to me."

The names and personal details of these two clients may change, but their stories aren't all that different. Both realize they can improve their lives by taking better care of themselves. The problem comes when they look solely to their bodies to give them the sustaining confidence or comfort they crave. Can you relate?

If so, welcome to *The Wellness Revelation.* It is awesome that you desire to improve your quality of life through better health and well-being. This book is designed to put you on that path, while helping you avoid the dead end that comes from missing this truth: Your Creator loves and values you as you are. As you seek to improve your physical fitness, He wants to free you from whatever is weighing you down. I'm not necessarily talking about pounds. I am talking about the "weight" that keeps you turning toward food (and neglecting your body) or turning away from food (and obsessing over your body). I am talking about the "weight" that comes from trying to keep life under your control. Are you stressed out and burned out? Then you have picked up this book at the right time.

Maybe you have struggled with your weight your entire life, riding a constant roller coaster of numbers that go up and down along with pant sizes. Or maybe you have recently begun to find yourself more stressed out and pressed upon by the world and all its demands. Perhaps you just don't feel as well in your body as you do in your spirit. The Wellness Revelation is going to change the way you perceive yourself and lay out strategies to improve your health. *This time* the change will occur from the inside out.

True confession: You could say I am a fitness dinosaur. I've been around since the prehistoric age of spandex leotards and Reebok high-tops. I went from participating in an early aerobics class in the mid-1980s to becoming a group fitness instructor in 1993. In 1996 I graduated from Arizona State University and went full-time into the fitness industry. I was in. All the way.

By 1998 I was the model of fitness with an award-winning physique. I had a successful personal training career and was newly married to a man who was going to take on the world. The money was rolling in, and on the outside, the package looked close to perfect. But on the inside, I was a sad, afraid, and miserable woman—desperate to be loved. I felt empty inside as I watched my marriage—not even a year old—nearly crumble under all the expectations I'd placed on it. Ironically, that void rested like a heavy weight inside me.

Enter Jesus: "Come to me, all you who are weary and burdened, and I will give you rest" (Matthew 11:28).

Around this time I noticed that Shawn, a fellow personal trainer at the gym, was changing. She was less rambunctious and no longer came to work exhausted and rough around the edges after being out late the night before. She was mild-mannered and laughed a whole lot more.

One day Shawn dropped a gospel bomb by walking straight up to me and asking, "Alisa, do you know Jesus?"

After I caught my breath and wondered if the separation-of-church-and-work police were going to show up, I stammered, "Yes."

"Great!" she said. "You should come to church with me!"

I quickly shot back that I couldn't go because my husband was not willing to go with me.

"So? You go," Shawn said.

Those three words hung over me like a physical fitness challenge, and I love a good competition. They haunted my sad heart for weeks. One Sunday I finally mustered up all the boldness I could and showed up alone and late to Shawn's church. After slipping into the back, I heard the gospel for the first time—even though I had heard it before. Jesus was right when He said, "Blessed are the poor in spirit, for theirs is the kingdom of heaven" (Matthew 5:3). In the past when I'd heard the Word of God, I hadn't felt like I needed Him. But now I did. I knew I was poor. I knew there was something going wrong within me, and the Good News could more easily seep into the cracks of my broken heart. That morning, it was as if the words Jesus spoke were just for me.

For the first time, I realized that as good as physical fitness felt and looked, it would not give me the joy, purpose, and rest I was looking for. Only Jesus could do that, and I found new joy and meaning as I began to follow Him.

Initially, I resisted the idea of my new faith and my fitness career somehow working together. Yet once I opened myself up to God, I began to see that my clients were longing for the very same things I had craved. Not only that, but God seemed to be inviting me to delve into His Word so that He could reveal His blueprints for healthy and whole bodies.

Finally, in 2007, my church graciously gave me space to begin offering a fitness class, called Revelation Fitness, which was open to the community. It quickly became one of the highest-attended outreach ministries on campus. Three years later, I launched an instructor training program to prepare others to lead fitness and wellness programs that would promote health and wholeness in their own communities. Revelation Wellness is now an international nonprofit ministry that uses fitness as a tool to spread the gospel message.

Through this book, we're inviting you to be a part of this fitness revolution. For the next eight weeks, you will move, step-by-step to the pace of grace, toward something greater than the number on the scale or the size of your jeans. You will learn the living and practical truth of what it takes to be healthy and whole (heart, soul, strength, and mind) while loving others as yourself.

Why does it matter? When asked what the greatest commandment was, Jesus said it was to "love the Lord your God with all your heart and with all your soul and with all your strength and with all your mind" (Luke 10:27). God asks us to love Him *completely*, just as He has loved us. Jesus then added that the second greatest commandment was to "love your neighbor as yourself." Loving others, however, is impossible if we are not fully connected to God, the source of pure love. After all, how can we love if we feel broken and disconnected from our true selves? That is why *The Wellness Revelation* is designed to help you renew the whole person, from the inside out. We will tackle the issues that matter most as you make complete and lasting lifestyle changes.

But here's the deal. If you desire *lasting* change, it's going to require you to:

1. *Show up.* This book is waiting for you. You paid for it not because you wanted to add another book to your stack but because you are hoping that *this* time, *this* book might offer the help you need. I believe it does. But just as if you spent hundreds of dollars for three weekly one-hour sessions with a personal trainer, that investment will pay off only if you show up. Every time you pick up and read this book, your personal soul-training session begins.

2. *Do the work.* There's no way around the universal law of reaping what you sow. You will get out of these eight weeks what you put into them. In each session, your spiritual and physical training will build upon the foundation you laid in previous weeks. To get the most from each session, you will need to:

   > Read: First, you will read the chapter for that week. This is a God-first book. Though it is packed with relevant information on diet and fitness, it wasn't created to tell you exactly what to eat and how to move. Instead, it was designed to enable you to develop fitness and nutrition plans that work for your life as you draw closer to the One who made you. As you seek God first, all the food- and fitness-related details will fall into place.

   > Respond: Many weeks include assignments to help you move toward improved health and well-being. Each week you'll also be encouraged to follow the Wellness Revelation Workout Calendar, available on

page 240 or at www.revelationwellness.org/book/workout. This eight-week calendar provides links to wellness coaching and fitness workout videos. Each Respond section opens with a brief explanation of what to expect from the activities on the calendar that week.

Throughout this eight-week journey, you'll be asked to move your body with a recreational state of mind. In other words, you will not move your body to pay off yesterday's calorie intake, or to pinch and prod your body into taking on someone else's idealized image for you. You are going to move your body as an act of recreation, believing that every time you move your body, the Spirit of the living God will meet you to shape and mold you into someone after His own heart. God re-creates when we recreate with Him.

> Renew: Every week you will also dig into God's Word, the only *true* source of renewal and transformation (see Romans 12:1-2). As you complete this section each week, you will allow the Word of God to train you and transform you into your whole and free self.

> Relate: Each week includes a number of questions that will help you apply the lessons and activities to your own life. Although you can do these on your own, I highly encourage you to partner with a small group or a friend or family member. As you exchange ideas and encourage one another, you will receive added incentive to keep moving toward your goals. It's been proven in the fitness world that the more accountability you have, the more likely you are to achieve lasting change.

> Reciprocate: Each week you'll read a true story meant to inspire you. As you begin to "weigh less," you, too, will be freed to help others carry their burdens—whether hunger resulting from the literal lack of food in a developing country or despair stemming from the lack of love,

peace, or meaning someone is experiencing closer to home. You'll read more about this below.

Be sure to access two additional resources throughout the coming eight weeks. The workout calendar, introduced above, will offer daily guidance as you begin developing healthy habits. The Moving Forward Journal, available for download at www.revelationwellness.org/book/workout, is a place to track your physical nourishment and movement, as well as your spiritual intake, for each day. This record isn't about earning your stripes, giving yourself a gold star, or shaming yourself when things don't go as planned. Instead, it will enable you to follow your progress and notice reasons to celebrate and give God glory as well as help you pay attention to any unhealthy habits you uncover.

3. *Be real.* You have to show up, do the work, and be completely you. Don't try to fake it for anyone else's sake. Don't live as if you have to audition for others' approval. Don't try to cover up your imperfections by donning another pair of spiritual Spanx. Our good God sees it all, and He is not offended by our messes. Achieving wholeness is possible only when we bring all of our insecurities and mistakes to the table. And we cannot heal what we are not willing to reveal, so please do yourself a favor and just be real. You are safe in His presence.

The life breath of *The Wellness Revelation* is the "exercise" of our faith. Weight loss and health gains can often feel like selfish endeavors, and sometimes they are entirely self-focused and self-driven. When we successfully reach our goals, we are tempted to take all the glory; when we fail to get what we want, we assume all the shame. That is one reason *The Wellness Revelation* contains one component that is missing from many fitness programs. As you "cast your cares on the LORD" (Psalm 55:22) and transform into a new being in Christ, your heart will be freed to help others in need. At Revelation Wellness, this is what we call "calories in" and "calories out"—receiving the fulfilling love of God (calories in) so you can give away His love to someone else (calories out). This is how the gospel message spreads! When you live in this way, you are running lean in the Spirit of God, relying on His love and power to bring hope, not only to yourself but to a hungry and thirsty world. The world is waiting for us to be "fit" for love!

During your eight-week journey, keep your eyes open for ways God may be calling you to serve others. Here are some ideas of how you might love others right where you are:

1. If you are completing *The Wellness Revelation* with a church body, what a blessing. There is power in agreement! Your group may decide to fund-raise and ask people to pledge toward your specific health goals. I highly encourage you not to make it about a number of pounds lost but to set more health-focused goals such as lowering your blood pressure, raising your whole-food intake, or lowering your processed-food intake. Perhaps your group could host a walk-a-thon while working through the book. Proceeds raised could go to a missions team or a family in need in your community. Or you might choose to complete a community service project as you go through the program together.

2. If you plan to work through this book on your own, I ask you to stop and go no further until you tell somebody what you are doing. Find accountability first; then, decide how you are going to love others. Look around and listen. Surely there is someone in need close by. Pray about it, and I am certain God will show you someone you can help as your own weights get lighter.

3. If you are taking this journey with a trained Revelation Wellness instructor, you are in very good hands. Each instructor is a God-first-and-foremost person and will be a great asset to you as you train according

to the Spirit and not the flesh. Your instructor can also advise you as you consider how God is calling you to love others. You are invited to go to www.revelationwellness.org/find-classes to locate a licensed instructor near you.

I know you may be thinking that you don't need one more Christian thing to do. You can be sure that I am not interested in adding to your load. But I do know that you are burdened, and some of that has to do with how someone has or has not loved you. You carry that weight in your body. If this describes you, your way of loving others might look like asking for forgiveness from someone you have hurt or giving forgiveness to someone who has hurt you. Perhaps for you, loving others will be less of an external service and more of an internal resolve to become increasingly patient and kind with God's help—a 1 Corinthians 13 kind of love. A love like Jesus.

Ralph Waldo Emerson is quoted as saying, "It is one of the most beautiful compensations of this life that you cannot sincerely try to help another without helping yourself." I couldn't agree more. That is the way of the gospel. You cannot outgive God's love. Giving helps you and me to be less self-absorbed; the more we spend ourselves on others, the more we receive so we can once again give it away. Even Jesus Himself said He didn't come to be served but to serve (see Matthew 20:28). Let's model our hearts after Christ's, opening them to continually receive and give away His love.

Please pause and consider that this eight-week process is going to take a commitment and a conviction to settle for nothing less than living the full and rich life that God intends for you. After all, you were created by God and for God because He loves you. He has a plan for your life, and He wants to free you up to live that life! I can promise you it will be better than anything you have ever imagined or dreamed, but it will come at a price.

There will be many moments of self-sacrifice and diligent work on your part. There will be times when you are tempted to turn back to your former comfortable ways. Hang on! Keep returning to hope. The payoff will be worth it.

In eight weeks, you will be gaining distance from your old self as you move closer toward your true self—a person who embodies God's love. Though the obstacles you and I face may differ, we are all on the same quest—to exchange old lies for truth and be set free. As you make this journey, you will be transformed and renewed, becoming more of the person you were truly meant to be.

EMBRACE GOD'S PURPOSE, DESIRE, AND DESIGN

Now to him who is able to do immeasurably more than all we ask

or imagine, according to his power that is at work within us.

EPHESIANS 3:20

Early in my fitness career, Karen, a more seasoned female trainer, told me that my body had great symmetry. She had quite the following among our clients, so I respected her opinion. Karen suggested that, with a little bit of effort and training, I could be a strong competitor in fitness shows. I was so hungry for meaning, validation, and approval that her words "You could be a real contender" were enough to make me look into what it would take to bring home a trophy from a competition.

For the next four months, I lost myself in the gym and spent hours in grocery stores looking for food to support my new goal of becoming a fitness champion. I read all the bodybuilding magazines and watched numerous fitness competition videos. I even enrolled in a beginners' gymnastics class filled with eight-year-olds so I could learn to do a back handspring—a necessary skill in the routine of any top-placing contestant. (Confession: I never learned how to do one. There's something about flipping backward that my twenty-one-year-old mind could not fearlessly approach. I even prayed that God would help me learn so I could place higher in all my shows, and then, of course, I would give Him some credit. God knew better.)

The final week before my first fitness show was sheer torture. I had to cut out carbs (the primary fuel for all the body's systems), eliminate salt, and continue trying to "cut" (or define) my muscles without destroying them. I felt as if I had the flu and wanted to punch everybody who crossed my path. I was miserable, hangry (hungry + angry), and irritable. It turns out that your body gets cranky when you aren't kind to it.

The night of the show, I couldn't have been more ready! With my skin painted the color of mahogany, oiled up to show the highs and lows of all my "cuts," clothed in my five-hundred-dollar purple competition bikini and Lucite heels, and with the number 15 on my hip, I walked onstage. I flexed. I did my quarter turns. Then I performed my three-minute, high-energy fitness routine (sans back handspring). A little later I came back onstage to hear the results. I was awarded third place. Although I had placed the first time I'd competed in a high-caliber fitness show, I didn't swoon and celebrate my accomplishment. I was focused on one thing: *Get me food!* As I walked offstage, I saw a disturbing vision that is *forever* burned into my brain. A fellow competitor who didn't place had walked off the stage before me. With a light sweat still glowing on her skin, she was kneeling in her blue bikini and heels before an Igloo cooler, shoving food into her mouth with animalistic fervor.

In that one quick moment, I was scared. It was as if I saw a neon warning sign over her head, flashing, shouting into my soul, "*Caution!* Danger ahead!" I wasn't walking with Jesus then, but I am confident He was walking with me. God was saving me—directing me from something that could have become self-destructive, not to mention obsessively time-consuming.

For me, fitness competing was playing with fire. God seemed to be telling me that if I made this my life purpose, I would not become the woman I was searching to be. Though I thought I could find purpose and validation by increasing my physical power and sculpting my physique, God, in His sweet wisdom and kindness, wanted to keep my heart from bondage and destruction. Even before I was faithful to Him, He was faithful to me.

GOD'S PURPOSE—HIS STRENGTH!

Though Karen's words had made me think I could find purpose by honing and showing off my own physical power, God had a better plan. In Exodus 9:16, He says, "I have raised you up for this very purpose, that I might show you my power and that my name might be proclaimed in all the earth."

God desires to show us His power and ability. We are to do *all* things in His power and in His way, not in our own. This includes weight loss and health gains.

His power strengthens us. What a relief! This means we are not on our own. Since His purpose is to show us His power and strengthen us through that power, we do not navigate our own course. To those who don't know God, this sounds like foolish talk. After all, we have a hard time relinquishing control. We grew up thinking that our goal in life was to become self-sufficient, productive members of society. We were taught that everything in our lives was based on our own accomplishments and life choices. We may have earned good grades, gone to college, graduated at the top of our classes, found good jobs, and lived morally upright lives, but still we wonder if it's enough.

As we embark on a journey to better health, it's tempting to tell ourselves that we just need to suck it up and be more disciplined, that weight loss and healthy habits are things we just need to "do." Before we begin beating ourselves up, though, let's ask, Is it possible that our choices, good or bad, could be a small part of a bigger plan that God can use for our ultimate good? Maybe these weight-loss, health, and body concerns are issues God can use to get our attention and gain our affection.

Desperation and disgust are powerful motivators for change, but they do not lead to lasting results and increasing joy. We ask for six-pack abs instead of a beer belly, when what we really long for is love. We ask for less jiggle when we walk, when what we really want is belonging without the fear of rejection. We agree to work harder, whether at our jobs or at the gym, when what we really hope is that our lives will have more meaning.

We were made for more.

For *The Wellness Revelation* to really transform our lives, we must soften our hearts. We need to remember our stories: where we come from and what God has already done for us. He has guided us every step of the way, planting and growing in us *His* purpose, *His* power, and *His* strength. God wants to remove the burden we carry when we think that everything hinges on our might and that the "win, lose, or tie" is all within our control. It is just not true. God desires to *be* our strength in *all* things.

God's power is made perfect in our weakness (see 2 Corinthians 12:9). For His strength to change us as we work through this program, we must surrender all of ourselves to Him. We *must* lay it all down with a humble heart.

HIS DESIRE—HOLY AND WHOLE

Once we've surrendered ourselves to God's strength and power, we organically develop a thirst to maintain unbroken fellowship with Him. Because outside forces will try to pull us away from His ways, we will always be in need of His sovereign and loving hand to guide our desires. Until people wanting to lose weight or live healthier lives understand this, they will continue to keep the weight-loss craze in business. Another book, infomercial, or unused treadmill (that will undoubtedly be used as a clothesline) will find its way into their homes and onto their credit cards.

How do we know whether we are desiring what God wants for us? Through His Word, He tells us what He created us to be.

First, God desires us to be holy (see 1 Peter 1:16). The Hebrew word for "holy" is *qadowsh*, meaning "set apart." The Greek word for "holy" is *hágios*, meaning "set apart from common use and dedicated to God." Sounds kind of snobby, huh? But being holy does *not* mean assuming that we are better than everyone else and should put on plastic bodysuits to keep ourselves from being soiled by others who just don't get it. What it *does* mean is that we "set ourselves apart" from what the world says is right and acceptable in order to follow God's will. He asks us to be holy (which involves doing things differently from others) for our own well-being, protection, and health so that we might protect, care for, and love others, glorifying God in all of it. Once we are called by God, we move from belonging to this world to belonging to the Kingdom where things are done very differently.

The Bible gives us all the direction we need to know how to act and live according to God's will, whether we are facing opposition, confusion, adversity, or celebration.

Scripture calls the process of moving toward holiness "sanctification." The pain that we go through, sometimes repeatedly, enables God to show us a doorway through our suffering. God meets us where we are, taking us by the hand and leading us through the fire. His purpose is always that we come out on the other side knowing the depth of His power and love. When we give ourselves to God, we will be sanctified (or set apart) from the ways of the world. Holiness (going a different way) is a by-product of our sanctification (letting God take us the better way). We begin to reflect a life like the one Christ lived—a holy and whole life. Christ in mind. Christ in heart. Christ in soul. Christ in strength. When we are holy, then we are whole.

God also desires wholeness for us. The dictionary defines *whole* as "containing all the elements properly belonging; complete . . . not broken, damaged, or impaired; intact . . . uninjured or unharmed."[1] Is that even possible? We all come broken, not whole, into this pursuit of better health. Our minds don't often reflect our desire to love God with all our hearts, minds, souls, and strength. In fact, this brokenness is what drives health and fitness trends. Humanity is seduced into desiring the perfect body (which, by the way, does not exist) so that we may reflect the image of perfection. Yet the one true image of perfection is found only in God. We were made in His image, and He is perfection. He lacks nothing. He contains all the parts and is not broken, damaged, or impaired. Through Him, our wholeness can be restored.

For the next eight weeks, we will be learning about and coming back to God's desire for us to be holy and whole. They exist together. The more we commit to God's way (holiness), the more whole we will become. This program is an opportunity to be put back together again by the One who made us and who knows where all the pieces go. He is the best psychologist, friend, personal trainer, life coach, and nutritionist we could ever have. God desires to come intimately near to us so He can reconstruct us to look more like Him. After all, this was His original plan: "Then God said, 'Let us make human beings in our image, to be like us'" (Genesis 1:26, NLT).

HIS DESIGN

If you question your value, remember this: You are God's design. In Jeremiah 1:5 He says, "Before I formed you in the womb I knew you, before you were born I set you apart." He personally formed you—every follicle of hair on your head, every cell of skin, and every unique quality that makes you *you*.

After preparing a world just for us, He "breathed" us into existence on the sixth day of creation. We are etched with the fingerprints of an awesome God! We are composed of intricate details that science has yet to figure out.

When I was in college, I loved taking art history classes. I was inspired by eye-pleasing art and was fascinated to learn the what, when, why, and how of each artist and his or her creation. I also discovered that understanding the artists themselves and knowing their experiences at the time they created a masterpiece led to a deeper appreciation for the designers and their work.

On a more personal level, you may have children in your life who've given you lopsided bowls from ceramics class, paper-cup ornaments for the Christmas tree, and macaroni bracelets and necklaces. When a child presents you with these creations, you wouldn't dare take them and throw them in the trash. They are beautiful in your eyes, and even more so in your kids' eyes, as they are the creators.

God is the ultimate Creator, and since He is never changing, we can discover in His Word more of what He might have been thinking as He designed us and breathed life into us. Have you ever heard the saying "How you care for the creation is a reflection of how you feel about the Creator"? Think about that. *You* matter to God. The *whole* you. That is why the way you take care of yourself— His creation—matters.

Currently, we face a growing epidemic in the United States (as well as globally). As of 2014, 70 percent of Americans were overweight,[2] and this number keeps growing. At the other end of the spectrum, some people engage in extreme bodybuilding (as I did) or have been trapped by eating disorders. Either way, too many of us are putting a lot of stress and strain on His design. From inside out and top to bottom, we alter ourselves physically, which in turn affects us mentally, emotionally, spiritually, and socially. We are no longer true reflections of His creation. We are not free to live and love as God originally designed us to. Let's get back to who we were created to be. You are His one-of-a-kind masterpiece. No other *you* has ever existed or will ever exist again. It's time to care for His creation—His design.

DESPERATION AND DISGUST ARE POWERFUL MOTIVATORS
FOR CHANGE, BUT THEY DO NOT LEAD TO LASTING
RESULTS AND INCREASING JOY.

RESPOND

With All Your Heart

> Be sure to access the Wellness Revelation Workout Calendar on page 240.
> This week you and I are going to meet via video, and together we will figure out
> where you are physically, in terms of muscle strength, endurance, flexibility,
> and cardiovascular ability. In a spirit of courage and kindness, we will find a starting
> point for your journey ahead. Don't worry or run away in fear! Tape measures
> and scales are not necessary. This will be fun—I promise!

MAKE A COVENANT

When you purchase a car, you sign a contract that solidifies your commitment to uphold your end of the deal by paying for the car. When you become a home owner, you sign a document in which you pledge to make your monthly payments. And when you commit yourself to another person in marriage, you sign a certificate that legally binds you to each other. Anytime two parties come into agreement concerning something of great worth, a formal contract or covenant is involved.

Covenant = "a mutual consent or agreement of two or more persons, to do or to forbear some act or thing; a contract; stipulation"[3]

Covenant (with theological implications) = "an agreement which brings about a relationship of commitment between God and his people"[4]

We were created by God for God, and each one of us belongs to Him. God purchased us back from the powers of sin and darkness through the blood of Jesus on the cross. As believers in Christ, we are now in a covenant, a love contract for life, with God Himself. Since we also desire to improve our well-being, something of great worth, let's get bold and make an agreement with God. Let's agree to let Him be God, and we will be His people.

On page 13, you will read and sign your covenant. I would ask that you find some quiet time to reflect, pray, and make this a moment when you put a stake in the ground. Place a spiritual marker in your life so you can look back and say, "That was when God did _____." Please sign the covenant and refer to it daily. May it remind you how faithful God is in carrying out His promises to you when you give Him your best yes.

YOUR ACTION PLAN

Most likely you have done some fitness goal planning in the past. This time I want you to make your plan by answering the following questions thoughtfully and intentionally. Be specific. (One-liners won't do.)

Please list your motivation(s) for choosing to complete *The Wellness Revelation* and the reasons you want to make a positive change in and for your health.

On a scale of 1 to 10, how motivated and willing are you to change? _____

What obstacles have kept you from making positive health changes in the past?

What are you willing to do in order to remove these obstacles?

List your top three physical health goals.

Example: *Reduce blood pressure so my doctor discontinues medication*

1. _____

2. _____

3. _____

List your top three spiritual health goals.

Example: *Grow in kindness toward myself and others*

1. _____

2. _____

3. _____

What are you hoping to learn from this experience?

THE MOVING FORWARD JOURNAL

You will begin keeping a food log this week (starting Monday), which is a key part of the Moving Forward Journal. You can photocopy the template on page 239 or download a copy of the journal at www.revelationwellness.org/book/workout.

I was inspired to name this journal Moving Forward by Exodus 14:15. After finally letting the enslaved Israelites go, the Egyptians had second thoughts and began chasing them down. As they approached the Red Sea, the Israelites feared for their lives. They cried out to Moses and to God. Moses replied, "Do not be afraid. Stand firm" (Exodus 14:13).

God told Moses in verse 15, "Why are you crying out to me? Tell the Israelites to move on." I love this. First, Moses directed the people toward God. The command was to not fear, but to stand firm in what they knew and trust that God would prevail. Then God directed them to *act*! It was as if He were saying, "What! Are you crazy? They are coming for you! Get moving. Put some feet to your faith." And as they moved toward the Red Sea, God parted it so they could walk across on dry ground.

That is what the Moving Forward Journal is all about. It will solidify your action plan to answer the call to live your whole life for God and others. This journal is designed to keep you aware of your thoughts and attitudes and to give you a place to record all your hard work, choices, thoughts, and feelings that are going into rebuilding your body, God's temple.

Your objective this week is simply to write down everything you eat and drink so that you can begin keeping track and being aware of the nutrients and hydration you're putting into your body. (If you have obsessed over food tracking in the past and have been afraid to be without your diet log or food apps so you can count every morsel of food and assign points, I invite you to break away from this habit. It could be mastering you and stealing your freedom. Feel free to use this journal for reasons other than tracking your food.)

Studies show that people who use some form of tracking tool to account for what they eat are more likely to lose weight and keep it off for as long as they continue to record. Don't worry: You will not be chained to a notebook for the rest of your life. I hope you will find strength, not in writing down your food intake, but in becoming more aware of what you are using to nourish your whole self.

You may begin making obvious changes to your nutrition, but you are *forbidden* (yes, I said it—forbidden) to swing in a radical direction to the point where you don't eat enough. Making extreme changes to your diet is a pride issue, which we will talk about next week. It has negative effects on your entire being.

The Moving Forward Journal also includes a space to record how much water you drink each day. Our bodies are about 60 percent water. Think of water as the oil that makes your engine run smoothly and cleanly. It is important that you get an adequate amount daily. A good rule of thumb is to try to drink at least half of your current body weight in ounces each day.

THE COVENANT

I, _____, choose to put God's desire and design
for my life first. I know that the Lord desires that I be holy and whole but that,
when separated from God, I break apart. I realize that I have neglected good
health in my life and the responsibility that I have in Christ to value such a gift.
This covenant proclaims that I henceforth am turning from my old ways toward
the new way. I acknowledge that hard work and sacrifice are to be expected, and
I will allow God to be my strength as I press on toward the goal. I understand that
this is a contract—an agreement—between God and me, solely based on love, and
I promise to make my health and wholeness in God a priority for His glory and
my joy.

    I promise myself that I will take the following actions as I give my whole
life—body, soul, and spirit—to Christ. Through the power of His grace, I commit
myself to:

> - showing up, doing the work, and being real;
> - staying accountable, first to God and then to my community of two or more;
> - partnering with faith and not with fear;
> - surrendering when I want to take back control;
> - resting in God's truth and His love for me;
> - seeking God first so that all other things may be added to me (see
>   Matthew 6:33);
> - knowing that God has made me on purpose for a great purpose;
> - letting God make and mold me, from my soul to my skin, into His
>   workmanship;
> - refusing to give in to shame or condemnation when things don't appear to be
>   going my way;
> - remembering—when I want to give up—that God's love never gives up on me.

Signature _____

Date _____

Perhaps your only change this week will be that you begin to write down what you eat and drink. That is enough. Don't worry about filling out the hunger scale or other elements in the journal now. They will be introduced next week.

In week 3 we will talk about reestablishing healthy and whole motives and purposes for physical activity. I know that might feel counterintuitive to some of you. Keep in mind we are doing things differently this time. In the next three weeks, through the use of your workout calendar, we will be intentional about getting you ready for healthy movement. (See the Wellness Revelation Workout Calendar on page 240.) While waiting to get to week 4, if you feel you would like to move your body as a joy-filled act, please do so. Just don't let your flesh into the driver's seat. Refuse to partner with a pinching or prodding spirit that is accusing and shaming you to "Move it to lose it!" That is not the voice of God. Shame is not part of God's training plan. Love is His eternal motivator. Move if you want, but only because love made you do it.

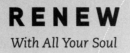

RENEW

With All Your Soul

The following questions are not meant to be a draining activity but rather an opportunity to set aside some disciplined and focused time to read, study, pray, and apply God's Word to your life.

His Purpose

1. Read Ephesians 3:20. What is God able to do? Describe a time in your life when you allowed God to be your power and strength. What was the outcome? How did that compare to a time when you didn't allow God to be your strength?

2. Read 2 Corinthians 12:9-10. What attitude should we have toward weakness? Why do you think God needs us to be weak in order for Him to make us strong?

3. How can we apply this concept of weakness when it comes to improving our physical health, which should make us stronger?

His Desire—Holy and Whole

4. Read Leviticus 11:44. What types of things keep you from living a holy life? What keeps you from living a whole life?

5. Now read Proverbs 14:12. Where do you see yourself following a way that "appears to be right" in your life? How might that be a stumbling block toward improving your holiness and wholeness?

His Design

6. Read Genesis 1:27. Since you were created in the image of God, what does your image say about Him?

7. Read Ephesians 4:22-24. What hope does this passage give you about how your life can be transformed in all areas, including your physical and spiritual health?

8. What deceitful desires corrupt your mind? (Keep in mind that *deceit* refers to something that misrepresents the real thing.) According to Ephesians 4:23, how do we rid ourselves of the desires that damage God's design?

Love Others

Prayerfully discern how God is calling you to love others during your Wellness Revelation journey into wholeness. Don't limit your thinking. Loving others doesn't always mean serving in a soup kitchen, knitting blankets, or volunteering at church. Sometimes, and dare I say usually, it means making that phone call and asking for forgiveness, or committing to risk loving someone who is not the easiest to love. To truly learn to love others, our weapons and walls must come down. Ask the Father what He is calling you to do. He knows, and He loves to tell you what is on His mind.

9. Please read Psalm 41:1-3. How do you see your commitment to love others impacting someone else's life? How might it impact your own?

10. In verse 3, the psalmist talked about restoring health. Where do you need restoration?

Dear God,

Through my weakness, Your power is made perfect. I invite You into my whole being and ask that I may know and feel Your strength. I ask that I might find power and purpose that I've never known before, which I can find only through Your loving grace. I desire to obediently respond to Your command that I be holy. I ask that You reveal Your path for holiness to me each and every day. Be my strength in the moments when I am confronted by any and all opposition to Your Word and ways. My entire body desires to be holy and whole. Heal me. Restore me. Please open my eyes to what You are doing, not just in me alone but in all of creation. I also pray for those who may be suffering, that I may rise up and be stirred to action. Help me see and do my part so that others may be healed and restored along with me.
✝ *Amen.*

RELATE

With All Your Mind and Strength

The following questions are designed to help you apply all you've learned this week to your fitness journey. Get with your accountability partner or small group and work honestly through these questions. Consider journaling your answers with God before sharing with your partner or group.

1. What does it mean to you to be *holy*? How would you describe it to someone who might not understand what the term means?

2. How is being holy connected to being whole?

3. Think about the most important relationships in your life. As you conform your life to holiness and wholeness, what might those relationships look like in the best of times and in the worst of times?

4. In the beginning, God created everything to work in perfect harmony. "God saw all that he had made, and it was very good" (Genesis 1:31). He made man and woman to live in perfect relationship with Him in a rich environment. Yet Satan, who'd once tried to take God's place, set out to

destroy humans' relationship with God by encouraging them to disobey the one command God had given them. Satan asked Eve, "Did God really say, 'You must not eat from any tree in the garden'?" (Genesis 3:1). After simply planting that seed of doubt, Satan watched as the first man and woman ate the fruit God had forbidden them to eat.

5. After they'd disobeyed the Lord, Adam and Eve felt shame over their nakedness. God asked them, "Who told you that you were naked?" (Genesis 3:11). The question wasn't meant to shame them but to invite them back into relationship with Him. Knowing that God wants to restore you to wholeness, too, apply this question to your own state of brokenness. Answer the question for yourself: "Who told you [insert a statement that caused you shame]?"

6. Adam and Eve sinned after they fell for Satan's lie and began wondering whether God was holding out on them. Take some time to write down the various lies that you have been living as truth—ways that you've believed God has been holding out on you.

RECIPROCATE

And Her Hair Grew Back

by Nadia Porter,
Revelation Wellness Ambassador*

I met Kate, at that time an addict and prostitute, while visiting a rough neighborhood with a team affiliated with the nonprofit Dream Center in a major city. Our team passes out roses and offers prayer to women like Kate who are struggling with prostitution and addiction.

When we first talked with Kate, we told her about the Dream Center and its three-phase program for women, which enables them to live at our facility, free of charge, for up to eighteen months so they can work on bettering themselves and preparing for a different occupation. In this seed-planting ministry, we typically do not see immediate results from our outreach. Occasionally, women choose to leave the streets and begin their journey with us; however, most of the time we only have the opportunity to pray over them.

Kate was an exception. In September 2015, she chose to surrender her life of addiction and prostitution and enter the Dream Center's program. Because I teach weekly fitness classes to women in the program, I was able to stay connected with Kate. During her first couple of weeks in my class, I watched her pale, tattooed body fidget with discomfort as I poured Scripture over her. Eventually, though, she came to know her identity in Christ and what it means to be a daughter of the Most High King.

As the weeks passed, her cold eyes became warmer and her shaved head began to grow beautiful brown hair. As she shared more of her story with me, it became clear that she was no longer the same woman—abused, shattered,

---

*Ambassadors have completed the extensive Revelation Wellness instructor training program and feel called to serve in low-income and marginalized communities to spread the gospel and move people toward healing and wholeness.

and hopeless—that she'd been when I met her. She was becoming whole and walking in more freedom than she'd known was possible.

I prayed constantly for Kate. Because the rules and class requirements of the program are incredibly strict, women often choose to leave the program before finishing it. However, all of those working with Kate were proclaiming a different destiny over her life.

In July 2016, I had a front-row seat to witness Kate's graduation from the second phase of the program. Through tears, I watched this beautiful woman with kind and compassionate eyes, long brown hair, and a smile that lit up the room tell her story from the stage to all in attendance, showcasing the glory, grace, and goodness of our heavenly Father. Kate had made it. By the grace of God, she had made it!

Kate is now finishing the third phase of the program and has integrated back into normal life. She has a job and an apartment of her own. I still see Kate every week, as she freely chooses to attend my fitness classes. She loves the way moving her body in worship makes her feel because it brings about a tangible change she can see and feel happening. She told me she is able to see how the Holy Spirit works in her through these movement classes.

One day, a woman named Marie began attending my class. She was shy and still felt quite sick, as her body was detoxing from drugs remaining in her system. She told me she was Kate's good friend from the days when they both worked on the streets. Marie explained that Kate had reached out to her and told of her experience in the Dream Center's program. Then she asked if Marie would like to surrender and begin a new life as well. Marie couldn't deny the change in Kate—she said she didn't even recognize her! Marie was not sure whether she was strong enough to make it through the detox process and the three phases of the program, but she agreed with me that the heavenly Father will give her the strength she needs. Marie is taking it one day at a time.

I stand amazed at the transforming work of Christ in Kate. She is no longer the woman she was, and not only that, she has now partnered with us by inviting women from her past to the program to change the darkest corners of this city for God's glory! Ephesians 3:20 says, "God can do anything, you know—far more than you could ever imagine or guess or request in your wildest dreams!" (MSG). What are your wildest dreams? Go on—dream bigger. Our God is a good Father who will fulfill the desires He placed in your heart. He will get His glory. Ask Him to do it; then simply stand back and be amazed.

BE FREE

Therefore, I urge you, brothers and sisters, in view of God's mercy, to offer your bodies as a living sacrifice, holy and pleasing to God—this is your true and proper worship.

ROMANS 12:1

As I was growing up, our home life revolved around two things: TV and food. Naturally, then, TV dinners were a key part of our weekly menu. God bless my parents! Like most Americans, they didn't know better. To them, these meals were just dinner. What could be so wrong about the blessing and provision of easy-to-prepare food?

When I was about fifteen, my parents allowed me to invite my best friend, Sali, to join us on our family vacation. Sali's family was very different from mine. They were the first family I knew who didn't own a TV, and they ate mostly fresh and healthy food. When Sali agreed to come on this trip, I knew it would be a very different experience, as my family's habits would be openly juxtaposed with hers.

During our weeklong vacation, we traveled to the California coast and visited Disneyland. On our way home, off the I-10 in Arizona, we stopped for our final feast at a local roadside McDonald's. We ordered our meals and sat down in a plastic booth. By this time, Sali and I were giddy from the long road trip. After a week of nonstop family fun, Sali was feeling right at home.

My father leaned over and asked her, "So, Sali, what did you think of our family vacation?" Sali grinned and said, "Well, I never knew you could make a vacation out of driving and eating." Of course we laughed, but that statement always stuck with me. It was the beginning of my eyes and heart being opened to the deeper questions about what my family valued. I saw the pitfalls of placing too much value on something that will never satisfy and ascribing value to something that has the power to steal from you. If you do, you will end up on autopilot, no longer paying attention and simply going with the flow.

What is it about food that always keeps us coming back for more? Well, of course . . . we *need* more because we need food to live. Part of the unique design of the human body is its need for food and its ability to enjoy food. That itself is a gift. God designed us so that we could eat and chew food (with our mouths and teeth), taste food (through our taste buds), break down food (using saliva, enzymes, and bile), and absorb and distribute food nutrients (through the stomach and small and large intestines).

It is all part of a deliberate and complete design. We are even told to pray for "our daily bread" (Matthew 6:11), whether it is physical or spiritual. Food sustains our physical life, just as the Word of God sustains our spiritual life. Throughout the Bible, we read how God used food to get His people's attention (through famines), to demonstrate His love and forgiveness (through the people's sacrificial offerings), and to enable His children to celebrate what He had done for them (through feasts).

Somewhere between Creation and now, our approach to food has gone seriously wrong. We have taken food and placed it in its own shrine. I have a shrine just down my street. You can't miss it. It appears almost holy—people even call it the Golden Arches, as if to compare it to the pearly gates. One thing is for sure: Eat too much of that food too often, and you might find yourself moving from the Golden Arches to the pearly gates!

When food—or anything, for that matter—is given the highest value in your life, it no longer serves you. You serve that which you give highest value. If food is the first priority of your life, it is actually malnourishing you and subtracting from your health while adding to your personal poverty. Looking back, I can see the emptiness my family was trying to fill with food and other material things that will never have the power to satisfy.

BONDAGE AND SLAVERY

Have you ever considered how easily we fall into the trap of "working for food"? We spend our time and energy thinking about food, preparing food, consuming food, and counting calories. An obsession with something other than God leads to idolatry—which traps us in bondage and slavery.

REMEMBER to use your Moving Forward Journal this week to track your food and water intake, as well as to remain focused on this week's Scripture verse. You can download a copy at www.revelationwellness.org/book/workout or photocopy the template on page 239.

Any good thing, like food, pain medication, wine, or money, has the ability to be used incorrectly. The enemy of our souls is placing bets that we will take something good and use it for selfish gain or pleasure. When we use something inappropriately, it gives birth to sin. The sin that starts out as "a little here, a little there" eventually grows into something that masters us—even as it seems to promise some payoff or reward. This is bondage. Bondage is involuntary servitude or, as it is more commonly known, addiction. Common examples of addictions are dependencies on caffeine, sugar, fat, and salt. You don't enjoy the payoff, but you keep returning to the addictive behavior because you feel trapped. You feel as if you have no will or choice, so you keep doing the very thing you don't want to do.

What starts as a necessary behavior (eating in order to survive) becomes more about the food and less about us—or about God, for that matter. And the payoff is no longer about sustaining life through the provision of energy. Eating becomes about the false high that feel-good food provides. The high is followed by the low. The need to assuage the low with the high creates bondage. "The high" becomes "the lie." When a food, substance, feeling, thought, or activity takes us captive, we are willing to stay chained to it in order to receive momentary payoffs. Food that makes us feel good can take us hostage and enslave us to a taste and/or a physical and emotional state that is tied to that specific food. We continue to stay in bondage, enslaving ourselves to a master (food) that has no plans to set us free, so we can get by for another day. And sometimes we unknowingly exchange one form of bondage for another.

Teri, a newly divorced thirty-five-year-old mother of two, walked up to me one day after I taught my spin class. She meekly asked if I would take her on as a client. Teri's face was heavy. Not in actual pounds, but in an "I haven't slept in weeks, I feel lost, and I am kind of scared to ask you for help, but I could really use it" kind of way. I liked Teri. I had noticed her as she'd quietly slink into class, weave between the tightly clustered bikes, ride hers with great focus, and then disappear from the room before all the usual post-class social shenanigans took place.

It just so happened that I had some time in my schedule, so a week later Teri showed up at my office for her initial consultation. She came in and sat down, fumbling around at first like a teenage girl on her first date. She knew that things were about to get really personal and that impersonal measuring devices were going to be involved. After some small talk, I asked Teri the usual questions: the goals she was hoping to achieve, the amount of time she could commit to a fitness program, and the obstacles that had gotten in her way in the past.

Teri made it clear that she was sick of feeling like a frumpy divorced mom and that her post-baby belly, eight years after the birth of her son, was no longer a welcome guest.

"Every time I drive my car and hit a bump in the road, I feel this jiggle!" Teri said as she scooped up a big handful of belly fat and shook it in great disdain. "It's like it's mocking me!"

By the time all the physical assessment and starting point measurements had been taken, Teri had the look—the tunnel-visioned, eyes-on-the-prize kind of look that says, "Nothing is going to stop me. This is going to happen. If you just tell me what to do, I will do it." The meek and lowly woman who'd entered my office in rayon work clothes and comfortable work shoes was leaving in spandex and a heart rate monitor, roaring like a lion. Teri was off and running toward the goal.

For the next four months, Teri never missed a session and never cheated on her eating plan. Her food logs were blue ribbon worthy. Three times a week she showed up, and not once that I can remember did she grumble or moan. She was the dream client. Change happened rapidly. Like, crazy change, crazy fast. In fact, I sensed that Teri might have been a little more restrictive on her diet than was healthy. But she seemed so content and energetic, not grumpy or tired (which you notice in most extreme restricters), that I didn't question her progress all that much.

Teri was happy. I was happy that she was happy. And the changes were undeniable. Teri was good for business. People in the gym were taking notice, and Teri was talking. Now some of her friends and family members were asking to meet with me. All was well.

Until there was no more to fix that could be pinched.

The problem was that Teri was beginning to see more and more issues to work on: "What about this part of my thighs?" she said as she pointed to the inner portion that seemed to jiggle a little. *That's called skin,* I thought to myself.

"Let's work on my abs a little more, can we?" she would often say. Teri was very afraid of that evil-eyed baby-belly monster returning.

Six months into our time together, I knew a transition was in order because things were getting scary for me when it came to Teri. As a former fitness competitor, I can tell you that Teri was as close to "show ready" as she could get without putting herself through one final hellish week of eating lettuce and dry tuna, dehydrating herself like beef jerky, and painting herself the color of cedarwood.

I asked Teri if we could do another assessment. I wanted to show her that she had reached a body fat goal that was far lower than the one she had initially hoped for. I wanted to assure her that she had arrived at her hoped-for destination and could rightfully celebrate and then enjoy the next phase of maintenance.

I will never forget the look on Teri's face after her final assessment. The numbers were lower than she had ever hoped for, and the before-and-after pictures were astonishing—jaw-dropping, in fact. As she sat in the same chair she had fumbled around in twenty-four weeks earlier, I looked at Teri and said, "You did it. Great job!"

But her eyes frightened me. They were vacant. And sad. She mumbled, under her breath, three words that still haunt me to this day: "So, that's it?"

"Yes. That's it. Now you can just maintain."

Teri walked out of my office looking like a fitness model on the outside but deflated on the inside. She left that day in the same way she used to inconspicuously slide in and out of my spin class, certain that no one could see her. I couldn't shake the sense that Teri went away feeling sucker punched and incomplete. In six months I watched her go from desperate to determined to disappointed.

Because we are all fallen creatures, we all, like Teri, are susceptible to bondage, which is the result of hardness of heart. Once we become enslaved to something for all the wrong reasons (sin), our hearts and minds lose their sensitivity to God. Over time, we become involuntary servants to food or whatever else has taken us captive. Bondage.

Remember, it is never about the food. The food is not the enemy. It is something deeper. Our relationship with food is broken because something deep within us is broken. God wants to heal us in those deep places!

Jesus came to rescue us. He can and will set us free! He wants to soften our hearts to make us sensitive to *all* things that cause pain and injustice (in our own lives and in others'). He wants to show us how to take pain, turn it on its head, and use it for good. He wants to make us more like Him, fit to be vessels of love.

God is *not* unfamiliar with bondage. As a matter of fact, He used a time of slavery to raise up a great nation. In the book of Exodus, we read about the Israelites, who, after the death of Joseph, began to multiply and grow in strength. The Egyptian king felt threatened by the Israelites and enslaved them, putting them under masters who oppressed them with forced labor (see Exodus 1:11).

Maybe something similar has happened to you. Without truly being aware of it, you have allowed your circumstances, experiences, and emotions (happiness, sadness, guilt, anxiety, inadequacy, stress, or fear) to be affected by your use or manipulation of food. The comfort or relief you initially felt after eating has become your payoff. However, it has left you feeling more depleted and chained to the endless cycle of addiction—serving a master who can't set you free.

IDOLATRY

You and I were made to worship. If we don't worship God, we will worship a false god: an idol (see Romans 1:20-23).

We often think of worship as the songs we sing in church, hands in the air, or on bended knee. But this is only one expression of the endless ways we can worship. Worship is adoring or ascribing total value to something, and we worship whenever we give ourselves totally to the thing to which we are devoted. When it comes to exalting God, our worship takes place in the biggest and the smallest acts, from prayer and quiet time to opening the door for a stranger. How we live our lives *is* our worship. We worship with who we are (our *being*—thoughts and feelings) and how we act (our *doing*—words, actions, and deeds). Yes, *every* aspect of life is worship.

Romans 11:36 says, "From him and through him and for him are *all* things. To him be the glory forever! Amen" (emphasis mine). All of life—our families, our jobs, our homes, our money, our food—comes from God through His sovereign power and endless love. The Hebrew word for "glory" is *kabod*, and it refers to something's great weight—whether literal or figurative. This *kabod* takes our breath away whenever we are near it. It is like standing next to the Grand Canyon. It is impossible to just walk by and not take notice.

Whatever we do, we are to do "for the Lord" (Colossians 3:23), and everything we do can point to Him, giving direction to others who are seeking a better way. That is one reason why what we choose to worship is so important. When we are worshiping God in *all* areas of life (health and vitality included), we are pointing people in the direction of this great wonder, so that they may also become breathless and inspired.

Romans 12:1 says, "I urge you, brothers and sisters, in view of God's mercy, to offer your bodies as a living sacrifice, holy and pleasing to God—this is your true and proper worship." In other words, our worship of God gives Him glory (affirming that all things weigh in His favor) and illustrates our dedication and willingness to sacrifice for Him.

The question is not *if* we will worship but *who* or *what* we will worship.

So what are you worshiping? What do you feel deserves your dedication and sacrifice of time, energy, and resources? If the answer to that question is anything other than God, you can be sure you are worshiping (giving your life to) an idol, a false god.

God is very clear on how He feels about us worshiping anything other than

THE QUESTION IS NOT *IF* WE WILL WORSHIP

BUT *WHO* OR *WHAT* WE WILL WORSHIP.

Him—and what happens when we do. The first commandment God gave us is "I am the LORD your God, who brought you out of Egypt, out of the land of slavery. You shall have no other gods before me" (Exodus 20:2-3).

The second commandment continues: "You shall not make for yourself an image in the form of anything in heaven above or on the earth beneath or in the waters below. You shall not bow down to them or worship them; for I, the LORD your God, am a jealous God, punishing the children for the sin of the parents to the third and fourth generation of those who hate me, but showing love to a thousand generations of those who love me and keep my commandments" (Exodus 20:4-6).

God knows that we *will* worship. If we do not worship the Creator (commandment one), then we will end up worshiping the creation (commandment two). We are living our worship of God when all that we do, say, believe, think, and feel points back to Him, showing our dedication and sacrifice for His glory—His *kabod*. When we no longer worship Him, we also break the second commandment and create an idol for ourselves.

Allow me to suggest some idols: food, drink, sex, entertainment, shopping, drugs, acquisition, competition, body beauty, nature, sports, family, children, pets, or a significant other. It is anything and everything that keeps us from wanting and loving God, dedicating and sacrificing ourselves to Him. Idolatry is when we think, *If only [fill in the blank with your greatest desire apart from God], then I will be happy!* Of course, these things never truly satisfy, and worshiping them leads us further away from God and deeper into depravity and despair.

In biblical times, people constructed idols when they sensed a need for God's presence. Instead of crying out to, relying on, and trusting God, the people created substitutes to fill their desire for the nearness of God. They spent time worshiping man-made statues or images. Each time, they sank further into ignorance and moral corruption.

There is only one God. There is *no* substitute (see Exodus 20:4-5). When we place food, drink, sex, drugs, etc. in the doorways of our hearts, we make it difficult for Him to enter. He prefers not to trip over the idols that we have placed at our hearts' doors. He desires to come into our lives, do some housecleaning, and reveal His power, purpose, and strength in us. Then He gets His glory and we receive our joy. Idols are a distraction, and our God is a jealous God. He is *not* jealous of the so-called gods we choose to worship; He is jealous for our love and adoration that we give to these cheap substitutes.

Has food become an idol that is hindering your love and adoration of your God? Is it getting in the way of your ability to love and value yourself as God loves and values you? Once you reach a point where food is no longer serving your good health, well-being, and Kingdom joy, you can bet you are serving food. It has you in bondage and/or has become your idol. Your good thing has become your god thing, and you are no longer free to abandon yourself completely to the worship of your Creator.

After God told Moses about His plan to free the Israelites, He told Moses to say these words to the ruthless Egyptian ruler who had enslaved His people: "This is what the LORD says: Israel is my firstborn son, and I told you, 'Let my son go, so he may worship me'" (Exodus 4:22-23).

Keep in mind that God was ordering Pharaoh to release his oppressive hand from the Israelites (His firstborn son). Moses appeared in front of Pharaoh six times and delivered God's message: "Let my people go, so that they may worship me" (Exodus 7:16; 8:1, 20; 9:1, 13; and 10:3).

Through this story, God shows us that we cannot fully worship Him, be totally available to His calling on our lives, and receive His abundant and freeing power when we are serving other masters and idols.

GLUTTONY

You know the old saying "Too much of a good thing is not a good thing"? So true! In our world, too much of a good thing seems impossible. We live in a culture where if a little is good, then *more* is better. We want everything to be faster, bigger, and better. Westerners are blessed to live in the land of plenty, but the land of plenty is slowly becoming a land of sickness and disease due to our overconsumption. Affluence and comfortable living breed false security, and with false security we fail to consider the ongoing impact of our comfortable lifestyles.

Gluttony is defined as habitual greed or excess eating. They are one and the same. Maybe your overeating habits started in childhood, when you weren't sure where your next meal was coming from. Out of uncertainty and perhaps anxiety, you ate and ate with abandon, ensuring that you got some food before it was gone. Maybe it was every man for himself in your home, and you ate simply out of a desire for more. Greed. Or maybe you lost rational thought when you saw a chocolate cake: If one piece of cake was good, then two were even better. Excess.

The Wellness Revelation is a battle cry for vigilance against greed and excess. It is a recognition that our excess has led to suffering—both our own and others'. It is an attempt to open our eyes to the injustice that surrounds us: the injustice that we (people who have) are dying from too much of a good thing, while others (people who don't have) are dying because we refuse to play a complete role in God's story—a role that would cost us our comfort.

THE TOOLS: FASTING

What the brain wants, someone once said, is often what causes it the most harm. In reality, we cannot trust our minds to know what is best for us. The brain will tell us it wants more sugar, salt, fat, or caffeine, but if we consume too much, our bodies will begin to rebel in the form of sickness or disease. When gluttony and addiction take root in our lives, we spiral from numbness toward death and away from *true* life.

We can, however, trust God's Spirit in us to direct us in the way we should go. He desires to break the chains of bondage, idolatry, and gluttony that hold us back. Fasting is a great way to free ourselves from being preoccupied with what *we* want. Fasting allows us to concentrate on our relationship with God and what *He* wants.

The Benefits

Physical

Our bodies were designed to rest from food periodically. Just as we are given the seventh day to rest from our busy lives, a fast is designed to rest the digestive system. One of the main benefits of sleep is its ability to rest and restore all the body's working systems. It is not an accident that the English named the first meal of the day "break-fast." Unless you are a midnight eater, you fast daily whether you know it or not.

God created our bodies and left His fingerprints of divine wisdom, mercy, and grace all over us, in hopes that we would find Him. When we pull a muscle, proper rest will help it heal. When we contract the common cold or flu, a day in bed will do us wonders. Your brain is wonderfully complex. Our Father is the Creator of all things, from the vast universe to the microscopic functions that keep us knitted together. He designed our bodies and our supporting systems to function best when they are given adequate rest (see Genesis 2:2).

When you eat, your body is forced to break down food into various forms of energy: carbohydrates, proteins, and fats. This breakdown process produces waste products. The cells have to clear this waste but can become overloaded. Fasting helps to free the system and eliminate the waste from it.

Fasting has also been proven to increase mental focus and calm our minds.

We know that food has a direct effect on how we feel, act, and think. It seems that given momentary breaks from food, our minds have the ability to achieve clarity and to remove the clouds that fog our mental focus. If we are honest, we often eat the food we eat, or do the things we do, out of sheer habit. We have lost our minds, no longer thinking about why we do what we do.

Habits that don't support us in living a healthy and wholehearted life are like stacked sandbags blocking the flow of a river that is meant to reach the thirsty ground of our hearts. In his classic devotional *My Utmost for His Highest*, Oswald Chambers suggested that believers make it a habit to have no habits. Even if we mean well in our lives for Christ, sometimes our best habits get in the way and keep us from serving Him with whole and pure hearts.

Fasting will allow you to cleanse yourself, for a period of time, from all positive and negative food habits. It will clear your eyes to see and open your ears to hear from God, the One who wants to be at the center of all that you do.

Please note: If you have battled an eating disorder like anorexia in the past, I would encourage you to take the idea of fasting before the Lord before deciding whether to fast. The enemy has stolen the power of fasting from you and twisted it into a prideful act of controlling calories by severely restricting food. But living by faith requires giving up control. As you seek God's will for you on this issue, I encourage you to ask God to remove your fear of losing control. If this is for you, He will give you a peace that transcends all fear.

Spiritual

The Word of God indicates that another benefit to fasting is spiritual healing. In Isaiah 58:6-8, God is upset with Israel for not truly fasting (with the right heart). He tells them that when they truly fast, "[their] light will break forth like the dawn, and [their] healing will quickly appear" (verse 8). Just as science validates that fasting produces physical healing, Scripture assures us that fasting also leads to spiritual healing.

Both the Old and New Testaments are full of examples of fasting. In the Old Testament, David fasted at the death of Saul (see 2 Samuel 1:12), during the sickness of the child born to him by Bathsheba (see 2 Samuel 12:15-22), and in prayer for himself and his adversaries (see Psalm 35:13; 109:24).

In the New Testament, Paul fasted following his conversion (Acts 9:9). The disciples fasted at the time of the consecration of Barnabas and Saul (Acts 13:2-3), as well as at the consecration of the elders of the early church (Acts 14:23).

People fasted so that they might hear from God. When we deny ourselves by fasting, we get out of the way so that God can take priority in our lives. We live in a world that wants us to believe that we deserve anything we want, but as a result we have lost ourselves. When we fast, we give Him the opportunity to be all that we need. When we humble and deny ourselves, we give Christ space to speak and move as only He can.

Not only that, but Christ Himself provided us with one of the most important examples of a fast when He abstained from food for forty days and nights. Right after Jesus was publicly baptized and the Holy Spirit descended upon Him like a dove, God opened up the skies to tell Jesus (and others who were listening) who He was: "This is my Son, whom I love; with him I am well pleased" (Matthew 3:17). Then the Spirit led Jesus into the wilderness, where Satan would tempt Him. Jesus went without food for forty days and forty nights, and He fought Satan with the Word of God (see Matthew 4:1-11).

His fast seems rather appropriate to consider in light of our focus on bondage. If you haven't faced some sort of temptation today, it is probably coming by the end of the day or maybe tomorrow. Either way, you can be sure it is just around the corner. Through fasting, we make a physical and spiritual decision that when we are tempted, we will be found standing with and for God. When we fast from our comforts, we are released from our chains so we can be found strong in Him.

Fasting for Poverty (Ours and Theirs)

Since we desire a revelation from God for wellness in our lives, a fast is in order. We fast not only to hear from God and get His perspective on our circumstances, but also to enable Him to develop our hearts and minds so they respond toward others as He does. We seek a godly perspective, not only on our own circumstances, but also regarding the people whom He asks us to care for. "For there will never cease to be poor in the land. Therefore I command you, 'You shall open wide your hand to your brother, to the needy and to the poor, in your land'" (Deuteronomy 15:11, ESV).

If you are currently overweight, it is probable that you have lost sight of what *true hunger* is. You might not even remember the last time you were *really* hungry. It is time to stop self-medicating with food! You need distance from your old ways as you turn toward the new. Fasting can be the catalyst for creating within you a new spirit and a clean heart for God, yourself, and others.

I'm not going to sugarcoat this. Fasting will make you uncomfortable. When discomfort from hunger arises, wouldn't it be powerful if you connected your momentary annoyance with those who suffer on an ongoing basis? What if you prayed for them and yourself? What a powerful moment of compassion that could be! If you sponsor a child in another country, mentor an underprivileged child locally, or see a homeless person standing on the corner with a sign, you could pray for him or her. So many around us suffer from poverty. Though some poverty is visible, the root of poverty comes from the hidden and unseen places, the places where the heart hungers.

Each time I fast, I am quickly reminded of how weak I feel without food. I understand how hopeless and ensnared by poverty those who don't have food must feel. We know that our food is just a few steps away in the refrigerator or a quick drive away at the local supermarket, while their next real meal could be days or even weeks away. Remember, God's heart is for the least. God has special concern for the poor (see Psalm 10:14-18). In the momentary, voluntary poverty of our fast, we reach out to their systemic poverty. I believe

God can bless this way of fasting, but only if it is truly our hearts' desire. Is it yours?

This is the fasting God loves:

Is not this the fast that I choose:
    to loose the bonds of wickedness,
    to undo the straps of the yoke,
to let the oppressed go free,
    and to break every yoke?
Is it not to share your bread with the hungry
    and bring the homeless poor into your house;
when you see the naked, to cover him,
    and not to hide yourself from your own flesh?
Then shall your light break forth like the dawn,
    and your healing shall spring up speedily;
your righteousness shall go before you;
    the glory of the LORD shall be your rear guard.
Then you shall call, and the LORD will answer;
    you shall cry, and he will say, "Here I am."

ISAIAH 58:6-9, ESV

RESPOND

With All Your Heart

> Be sure to access the Wellness Revelation Workout Calendar on page 240. This week's videos will guide you through your remaining health assessments. If you are beginning to feel like this fitness pace is too slow, notice that this is your flesh trying to take the reins once again. Remember, "Love is patient, love is kind" (1 Corinthians 13:4). This wellness adventure is about Love having His way in you.

STEP ONE: THE FASTING ASSIGNMENT AND HUNGER SCALE
Fast

If you hear nothing else, hear this: *There is no lasting benefit to a fast unless it is accompanied by a spiritual hunger.* Please do not enter this fasting assignment lightly. If you are not feeling hungry to hear from God on the matter of your health, it may be best that you skip this assignment for the week. When you fast, your motivation cannot come from a prideful heart. It must come from your desire to seek God and hear from Him. Take some time to pray about it and see if your spirit is prompting you to fast. Fasting just to fast is a religious act, and we aren't seeking more religion. We aren't seeking to do acts for God to earn His favor. We are simply seeking Jesus and the freedom that comes from drawing close to Him.

You are invited to do a standard fast—abstaining from food for a defined period of time. How long you fast is less important than how willing you are to let God lead you in and out of a fast. It would be best not to set out to meet some predetermined goal based on time. Make hunger for more of God your goal.

As you prepare for and engage in your fast:

1. Please be sure that you set aside the right days to fast. In other words, if you have never fasted before, it is probably best to fast for one day, and plan it for a time that you know will not conflict with work, school, or family in a stressful way. Personally, I find fasting from dinner on Saturday to dinner on Sunday a perfect time. I know that on Sunday I will be resting all day and feel no need to do anything in particular, other than to live with a grateful heart. Pick the time of your fast according to your schedule.

2. While fasting, take intermittent times to talk with God, especially when hunger pains or the desire to eat arises. When tempted, go to a quiet place, open your Bible, consume (eat) God's Word, and then pray. This is a good time to ask Him questions about His heart for you and for others. Your mind is freeing itself from the chemical reactions that come with metabolizing food, so be excited about the mental space that you are creating and allow the Lord to speak to you. Your "house" (heart and mind) is being cleansed, also known as detoxing. What better time to read God's Word and to talk with Him in prayer! This is the good stuff! In our weakness, His Word shows itself strong and comes to life.

3. The minute fasting becomes too much and you are not able to find peace from prayer, or you are no longer motivated by a desire to connect with God, it would be best to end the fast. Fasting should never be about what you can do for God or about your own pride. Stay hungry to connect and realign. When you can't seem to settle yourself in the Lord's presence, end the fast and move to step two of this week's assignments.

4. Drinking water is encouraged, and drinking juice if necessary is acceptable in a standard fast.

5. Be sure to journal about your experience. Write down and record whatever God might be revealing to you during this time.

6. Expect mild symptoms like headaches, weakness, or irritability. Other symptoms may include bad breath, frequent urination, sleeplessness, or a sensation of feeling cold. The severity of your symptoms might depend on the degree to which you suffer from food addictions.

7. Be of good cheer! Remember Jesus' counsel about fasting: "When you fast, do not look somber as the hypocrites do, for they disfigure their faces to show others they are fasting. Truly I tell you, they have received their reward in full. But when you fast, put oil on your head and wash your face" (Matthew 6:16-17). Don't walk around looking sad and asking for pity because you "can't" eat. Don't get trapped into thinking how strong you are for not having to eat. Have a smile on your face and be joyful about what the Lord is doing in you and through you. He is yours and you are His!

The Hunger Scale

Once you have broken your fast, you will begin using your Moving Forward Journal in more depth by rating your hunger. The hunger scale is designed to rate hunger on a scale of 1 to 5:

1. Very hungry: You likely are experiencing a headache and crankiness. You feel tired and run down. You should feel this when ending a fast and only when ending a fast.
2. Hungry: You feel a small ache, discomfort, and grumble in your stomach.
3. Content: No need for any food at this time.
4. Satisfied: After eating, you feel satisfied. You ate only what you needed.
5. Gluttonous: You crossed the line and ate more than your body needed. You feel uncomfortable in pants that don't have an elastic waistband.

During the remaining six weeks, you will rate your hunger before you eat and after you eat in your Moving Forward Journal. You are encouraged to do this with every meal and snack. Note that you will probably shift back and forth between a 2 and a 4 throughout your day. This is normal and relates to a healthy blood sugar level as well as a healthy metabolism. By learning to be more aware of hunger and how it relates to your eating habits, you will be changed *by* God and *for* God.

Be sure that you are eating due to hunger and not out of boredom or mindlessness. It's possible you will reach a level 2 between meals and need to refuel to a 4. My hope is that you rarely or never experience a 1 or a 5 during this time of retraining your habits. This hunger scale is going to play an important role in creating a sense of consciousness about when, what, and how you eat. Weight gain often occurs when we have checked out; we have stopped paying attention to whether we are truly hungry or are eating out of habit rather than hunger.

Taking time to rate your hunger before and after eating will begin to train you in the practice of mindfulness, and that mindfulness will carry over into all aspects of being holy and whole.

STEP TWO: USE ALL PARTS OF YOUR MOVING FORWARD JOURNAL

Last week you began recording your food and drink in the food log portion of your journal. Beginning this week, you will also complete the hunger scale (see above) and the other sections of the journal:

1. *Bible verse.* Each day, at the top of your food log, you will rewrite the Bible verse found at the beginning of that week's opening page. (For example, week 2's verse is found on page 23.) Each verse pertains to the main topic for that week, and writing it out will help it soak into your mind every day. It will become your *life verse* for that week.

2. *Prayer/devotional/quiet time.* Your prayer and devotional time can be done in conjunction with reading and meditating on our weekly Bible verse.

When we pray and become quiet before God, we are taking time to put God first—to be inspired. God is always speaking, but we are not always listening. Finding a quiet place and being still before God requires a lot of discipline. We can always think of other things we could be doing with that time, but they will never pay us back the way time with God can. We rarely finish a workout saying, "I wish I hadn't done that." Likewise, we will never walk away from our time with God wishing we hadn't done it. It is always nourishing. We *always* feel stronger and more energized afterward.

The Wellness Revelation is a springboard to a holistic life. This means we seek spiritual obedience so we can have physical discipline. Remember that God is our strength for this. Choose a good study Bible or daily devotional as your tool for this extended quiet/devotional time.

When you sit down to have a quiet time, take a few deep breaths. Find a place of quiet on the inside and, most importantly, try to set aside all your wants and desires. Pray that God will direct you to what He wants you to read for that day and that you will let the words read you! Pray that the Word will come alive so that you can live it out that day and in the days to come. If you are going through tough circumstances, temptations, or moments of weakness, ask God to meet you there. Pray that He would speak to you right where you are. Be patient. God's timing is perfect.

Once you've committed this time to God, I encourage you to engage in a wonderful ancient form of meditation on Scripture called *lectio divina*. This is a way of reading Scripture and meditating on it so that it changes you from the inside out. Don't read these daily verses as you would read a textbook. Yes, they are truths and facts, but I pray that you will allow the words to go beyond the surface level of your comprehension and deep into your soul. May the words you read bring new meaning and life to the quest for a healthier you. Try out *lectio divina* with these four steps:

> Eat the Word: Instead of just reading the Word, I would ask that you "eat" the Word. In other words, read slowly and thoughtfully several times, fully digesting and consuming the Word so that it saturates your soul and breaks down, as food does, to nourish every part of your spiritual being.

> Think: Spend some time thinking about what you have just read. What word, phrase, or sentence piques your interest? Study that word or concept a little deeper or journal further about what you sense God is saying to you about it. This is when the mind begins to renew itself. Also, resolve to continue thinking on that word throughout your day, especially in overwhelming or stressful times. Come back to that Bible verse and meditate on it, if only for a minute. Let your mind carry the Word into the unexplored caverns of your consciousness. Who knows what might come forth and inspire your soul?

> Pray: Talk to God about what you just spent time thinking about. Praying about the Scripture invites the Holy Spirit to translate it for you. When you pray, you enter that holy place where your soul can find peace. You can ask for further insight into your reading or just rest with whatever impression God gives you through the feeding of His Word. Prayer is simply talking with God. Just as in any relationship, the two-way street of talking to be heard and listening to understand only strengthens your connection with Him.

> Live: Finally, go out and live the Scripture. Don't leave God behind in the pages of your Bible, but be sure that you give Him opportunities to use that piece of Scripture sometime in your day. Be ready and able to draw upon the sword of the Spirit (the Word of God) when the battle arises.

3. *Food log.* Last week you began recording your meals, snacks, and drinks. What you eat and drink is just as important as how you think and feel.

I hope the Moving Forward Journal will provide you with an outlet to reflect upon your choices. Writing things down when taking on a new health endeavor can be helpful for addressing plateaus or sticking points that threaten your progress. We will talk about food choices next week.

Disclaimer: If you constantly count calories and are consumed by what you eat, you are not to log your food. It's time to take your eyes off the notebook or the calorie-counting website and put them on the only One who counts—God. I do encourage you to use all the spiritual training features of the journal.

4. *Drink log.* It isn't necessary to force hydration, but if you are used to drinking primarily soda, coffee, and tea, you are probably very dehydrated. It may be a challenge for you at first to get your body back to a healthy level of hydration. Up to two thousand pollutants and chemicals can be found daily in your local water supply (tap water), so make sure you receive your water from a pure source. Most people think bottled water is a good choice. Bottled water is regulated by the Food and Drug Administration, but unfortunately bottlers only have to pass certain standards once a year. A home filtration system provides the best water.

STEP THREE: SLOW DOWN!

Seeking God before doing anything in life affords us the opportunity to take our needs to Him first and ask Him to be our Sufficiency. We know that in our own might and wisdom, we are sure to fail. Praying before eating is not just about blessing our food or performing a ritual. Praying is about acknowledging the blessing of our God and all that He has done for us in this moment and throughout the day. I am convinced that if we take the time to pray before we eat, we will see a change in how (and how much) we eat.

Rather than thinking of it as saying grace before your meal (which can, at times, seem ritualistic and lifeless), how about approaching prayer like breathing before you sit down to eat? Breathe to center yourself before you take that first bite, so that you don't eat *mindlessly*. Praying and breathing before eating is like slowing down at a speed bump before reaching the plate. In this hurried world of fast-paced "go-go-go," who has time to pray? I will tell you who. If you want your mind renewed and your body transformed, take *all things* to Him before acting.

> Seek first his kingdom and his righteousness, and all these things will be given to you as well.
> MATTHEW 6:33

During this journey together, I ask that you try to develop a studied, practiced, and merciful prayer life. Every time you put a plate in front of yourself, slow down and gently go over the speed bump before you take your fork to your mouth. First, take a few deep breaths. Deeply inhale and then deeply exhale, even longer than the inhale. Refrain from praying until you find you are less anxious. Then pray a centering prayer, perhaps something like:

Dear God, I thank You for the supply of food that You have placed before me. Because You are my Sufficiency, I ask that You give me the patience and focus to take each bite and savor the gift so that I may stay conscious and mindful. Allow this food to give my body just what it needs. Take this food and transform my heart, mind, body, and soul to be more like Christ. Amen.

Or even:

Jesus. Thank You. Sit with me. Eat with me. Amen.

Remember, prayer takes place in the heart, not in the mouth. The words you say do not matter. What your heart says does!

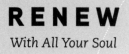

RENEW

With All Your Soul

S et aside some disciplined and focused time this week to read, study, pray, and apply God's Word to your life.

Bondage/Slavery

1. Read Exodus 2:23-25 and 3:7-10. What were God's reasons for rescuing the Israelites from their slavery? How might these passages apply to your current circumstances with health, weight, or food?

2. You might argue that what God did for the Israelites does not pertain to your current struggles: "God doesn't know the struggles I face today. That happened over four thousand years ago. What does that have to do with me today?" Read Exodus 3:11-14. Pay close attention to verse 14. Based on that verse, what can you be sure hasn't changed since the days when God rescued the Israelites? How could you allow Him to fulfill His purpose in your life— to be your strength and your center—today?

3. According to Exodus 13:3, what did it take to free the Israelites from their bondage?

Idolatry

4. Read Romans 1:21-25. What can happen when you know of God but refuse
    to let Him be your God?

5. Why do you think people exchanged the glory of the immortal God for
    images of mortal humans and animals? Keep in mind that people created idols
    in order to feel close to God, to connect with Him, or to fill a need. Have you
    used food or other substances in this manner? Be specific. Detail a time when
    you can clearly remember using a substance such as food for fulfillment.

6. What does Galatians 4:8 have to say about slavery and idolatry? My prayer
    is that through the Wellness Revelation, you will begin to know the true and
    real God better than ever before. May He show you His unbridled strength
    and love. May you never feel another need for a substitute, and may you
    hunger only for the real thing, which is Christ.

Gluttony

7. Read Philippians 3:18-21. Pay particular attention to verse 19: "Their
    destiny is destruction, their god is their stomach, and their glory is in their
    shame. Their mind is set on earthly things."

    Fill in the blanks: "Their destiny is destruction, their _____
    is their stomach, and their _____ is in their shame." What
    happens when we set our minds on earthly things?

8. What does Proverbs 23:20-21 have to say about gluttony? *Gluttony* means "excess in eating or drinking." How is it that poverty can result from gluttony?

9. Describe, in greater detail, the poverty in your own life. (Poverty can be defined as relationships that don't work, whether spiritual, physical, emotional/intellectual, or social.)

10. How might your relational poverty be similar to the experience of people who live in developing countries? (There is no wrong answer; invite the Holy Spirit to help you be creative and thoughtful with your response.)

God,

Help me to understand what You are doing in my life. As You begin to peel back the layers of my life, You are showing me the places where I have failed to let You be God—where I have tried to make a good thing my god thing. From a humble heart, I desire to seek You. You are my God. You are I Am. I admit that I am fearful of letting go of the things in my life that are taking Your place. I fear loneliness, sadness, and weakness. I believe in the promises You have made, so I can be free to love and be loved by You alone. Please continue to lead the way and give me Your strength to follow.
✝ Amen.

RELATE

With All Your Mind and Strength

The following questions are designed to help you apply all you've learned this week to your fitness journey. Get with your accountability partner or small group and work honestly through these questions. Consider journaling your answers with God before sharing with your partner or group.

1. To discover your idols, ask yourself the following questions: What do I fear most? What do I love most? Or finish this sentence: "If only [fill in with any circumstance, want, need, or thing], then I would be complete." Write your responses below.

2. Did you fast this week? Why or why not? If you did fast, how did it go? What, if anything, did God reveal to you?

3. Did you experience true hunger coming off the fast? How did that affect your awareness of your eating patterns and habits?

4. Are you using the hunger scale now? If yes, what are you learning about your hunger? If you are not using it, why not?

5. How are you feeling about your food logging? What are you learning?

RECIPROCATE

Finally Free

by Vivian Hall,
Revelation Wellness Instructor

I met Mary when I led a Revelation Wellness fitness class in a women's prison. I learned that she had grown up in a middle-class family. She attended church and remembers saying the salvation prayer when she was four years old. Mary told me her family was happy until her parents divorced when she was twelve. After that, she lived with her mom, and she no longer went to church.

Her mom remarried, and Mary had a very good relationship with her stepfather. Then when Mary was fifteen, divorce devastated her life for the second time. Through that loss, many wounds formed in her heart. Depression, a sense of abandonment, and the deep need for a father figure caused her to turn to men out of desperation. Soon she was involved with a bad crowd and began using many kinds of drugs. At age sixteen, Mary was kicked out of her house and began living with a boyfriend. Even so, she graduated high school with honors and then earned a bachelor's degree in graphic design. On the outside, Mary looked as if she had it all together. However, she began to use drugs again and learned to hide behind her success. Mary became addicted to prescription drugs, and her life spiraled out of control fast.

Addiction to amphetamines began to run her life. She committed several crimes to feed her habit. She was in and out of prison, serving a few years each time. During Mary's last stint at a women's correctional facility, she joined a therapy program, began to get some healing, and grew close to the Lord again. She started to attend church services as often as she could and finally learned to build her recovery on the foundation of Jesus Christ.

One day Mary received a flyer about a new program that was coming to the prison—the Revelation Wellness class I was leading. She was so excited! She loved that the flyer said to love God first and worship Him through fitness. He was now number one in her life, and her love for fitness made her curious about a class that would combine faith and fitness. The word *wholeness* on the flyer stood out to her the most. After applying, Mary couldn't wait to find out whether she was going to make the cut to be in the class or if she would be put on the waiting list. She was so excited when she made the cut!

When Mary attended her first Revelation Wellness fitness class, the experience was indescribable. She told me she felt the supernatural power of the Holy Spirit. She looked around the room at the other women and could see the transformation on their faces. She was hooked! The next week, Mary spoke to me about becoming a Revelation Wellness instructor herself. I encouraged her and said that I would get her information on how to sign up. The week before she was to leave prison, I brought the training material to class. Mary shared her passion with everyone, and we prayed for her.

When Mary was released from the correctional facility, she went directly into a strict work release program. She worked sixty-five hours a week, stayed busy attending church and serving others, and continued her recovery work. She plans to become a Revelation Wellness instructor when the time is right and to use the training however the Lord leads.

LIVE OUT HIS PURPOSE FOR YOU

"Everything is permissible for me"—but not everything is beneficial.
"Everything is permissible for me"—but I will not be mastered by anything.

1 CORINTHIANS 6:12

When I was fourteen, my new friend Julie invited me to an aerobics class. This was three years after Jane Fonda released her first workout video, so everyone was aware of the leotard/banana hair clips/scrunchie sock look from TV. To a certified tomboy like me, though, aerobics seemed exotic, and the thought of moving my body in an organized fashion was intriguing and intimidating.

But why not? I thought. *I'll give it a go.* I didn't have the official workout duds (no spandex leotard or shiny flesh-colored tights), so I figured a cotton T-shirt, my gym shorts, and some K-Swiss sneakers would have to do.

As soon as Julie and I walked into the newly opened aerobics studio in the strip mall, I was blinded by the spandex. The colors. The high-stacked, hair-sprayed, permed hair held back by terry cloth headbands. The instructor, Jackie, a tall, beautiful African American woman with strong legs, toned arms, and a bright smile, quickly put me at ease. She clapped her hands and shouted, "Okay, ladies! It's time! Let's get moving!" My heart began to race in excitement and fear of the unknown.

Jackie walked over to the corner, pulled out a vinyl disc, placed it in the record player, and then dropped the needle on the record. *Boom!* Like a freight train, we were off—doing jumping jacks, aerojacks, grapevines, and rocking horses. I was picking up a new language, set to the *Blues Brothers* sound track, rather quickly.

I loved every single moment.

For that one hour, all the fears and insecurities I had as a typical teenager seemed to be swallowed up in a chasm of joy. I felt free. I felt like I could do anything. I had a sense that joy was my birthright.

At the very end of the class we lay on the floor on our backs, like scattered corpses. Instead of feeling dead, I had never felt more alive. As we lay there, Tracy Chapman's "Fast Car" playing in the background, Jackie walked between us, speaking softly.

"Well done, ladies. Remember to breathe now. That's it—just a gentle stretch."

As Jackie's kind words reached me, a thought crossed my mind. It was unlike any other I had ever had. *Whatever that woman just did, I am going to learn how to do that.* I now know with certainty that this inspired idea did not come from me. It was the beginning of discovering my life purpose—to lead others into a life of joy and freedom. Though it would be years before I led my first workout session, I had found my work assignment.

We commonly use the word *vocation* to describe our life's work. The root word, *vox*, means "voice." Without realizing it as I lay on the floor of that aerobics studio, I had also found my voice.

God created you for this world, here and now, to speak into the world in a way that only you can. Your voice—your work—is as unique as your thumbprint.

Even if you find yourself burned out, worn down, unexcited, or drained from your current life's work, I have great news: God can bring new life into old work—*your* work of everyday living—and free you from the "blahs" of the daily grind.

Our lives are about glorifying God and giving Him a good name. As Paul states in 1 Corinthians 10:31, "So whether you eat or drink or whatever you do, do it all for the glory of God." That is our work!

We have the opportunity, as we simply go about our everyday lives, to do work as a witness. We provide evidence that Jesus is who He says He is: our Redeemer, Savior, Helper, and Encourager. This sums up God's work, which He does every day without ceasing. He saves, helps, encourages, and loves like no one else ever could.

When people look at you, do they see this power of Christ in you? *We*

REMEMBER to use your Moving Forward Journal this week to track your food and water intake, as well as to remain focused on this week's Scripture verse. You can download a copy at www.revelationwellness.org/book/workout or photocopy the template on page 239.

---

display God's glory to others. With our lives, we proclaim that He is our Strength and that He picks us up out of the pit to release us from bondage. Then we exhibit His strength through the choices we make, the actions we take, and the voices we use. What we do with our bodies, whether it be a hug or a handshake, a push-up or a push away from the table, shows Christ's love and power inside of us to a world that needs to see this great mystery.

When writing his first letter to the Corinthian church, Paul said a lot about how the believers there used their bodies. After all, the temple of Aphrodite (goddess of love), with more than one thousand temple prostitutes, dominated the city of Corinth. Paul reminded the believers there that their bodies were the temple of the Holy Spirit. Our bodies do not belong to us, and we are to honor Christ in the way we use them (see 1 Corinthians 6:19-20). We can't authentically bear witness to Christ if we treat our bodies in contradiction to His ways.

Brennan Manning, a great author, former priest, and speaker who for many years struggled with alcoholism, is credited with pointing out that "the greatest single cause of atheism in the world today is Christians who acknowledge Jesus with their lips then walk out the door and deny Him by their lifestyle. That is what an unbelieving world simply finds unbelievable."[5]

We have a calling to be authentic in our life's work—to live out our vocation so that God the Father, Christ, and the Holy Spirit receive glory, honor, and fame. That includes how we care for our bodies. As I stated in week 1, 70 percent of Americans are overweight, with nearly 38 percent of those people facing morbid obesity.[6] And those percentages are going up. The number of people affected by this epidemic is rising, with the diagnoses of heart disease, insulin-dependent diabetes, high cholesterol, and high blood pressure also increasing.

As the church, we have an obligation and a great opportunity to *be* the change. "For the Spirit God gave us does not make us timid, but gives us power, love and self-discipline" (2 Timothy 1:7). We are called to live for a higher purpose, which calls us to higher accountability and self-discipline. If others see us living in poor health and disease while filling ourselves with things that don't help but hurt our health, what are we really saying about our God of power and love?

What do you think when you read the word *self-discipline* above? I am not surprised if it leaves you feeling burdened. After all, you didn't choose many of the sharp pieces of your life's puzzle. Maybe you've faced divorce, depression, betrayal, or loss, and you've turned to food or other addictive substances instead of turning to God. You may have taken the puzzle pieces of life and tried squeezing them into the wrong places to make them fit.

When it comes to our goals for changing ourselves, we often try harder at working our plan. In fact, this approach is rampant in the weight-loss world. I want you to exhale because we are about to flip that idea of self-discipline on its back and pin it to the mat. I want to give all of us a new way to look at self-discipline, also known as self-control, which is one of the fruits of the Spirit (see Galatians 5:22-23).

This doesn't mean living perfectly. That is far beyond us. It does mean living in the truth that God is love (1 John 4:16). That realization leads to wholeness: living as who we are—dearly loved, valued, and cherished children of God who happen to live in a fallen world. We look to Jesus, whose purpose in coming to earth was to exhibit the power, love, and grace of the Father. He faced the same struggles, trials, and temptations that we do but stayed pure in heart, mind, and body. He was blameless. He is the embodiment of the God-reality that a purpose-filled life is one that is *holy* and *whole*.

In response to His love, we desire to follow Him. Our obedience is a natural overflow of our love for God: "If you love me, keep my commands" (John 14:15). The more you know who God is and who you are in relationship with Him, the more you will grow to love Him. The more you love Him, the more naturally obedience will come. So the root of obedience—doing whatever God asks in order to live in agreement with His purposes—is love.

Obedience precedes self-discipline. Obedience trumps self-discipline. Obedience is the cause, and self-discipline is the effect. And according to Jesus, obedience is something that we will desire because it feeds our love affair with God. People who love God look the temptation of eating another cookie or obsessing over their bodies in the eye and say, "Get behind me. I have something so much better than you."

LOVE AND ENERGY: THE ABILITY TO DO WORK

Besides centering your being and doing in God, what is needed in order to complete work? Energy!

Food is the fuel that produces the physical energy we need to do our work. Just as God has a plan and a purpose for us, He also has a plan when it comes to food, drink, and nourishment for our bodies and souls. Food gives us the energy to do *His* work—the work of loving and living well. Mercifully, God's part is to do the work in and through us. Our job is to care for ourselves today by making choices for our health that will benefit us tomorrow.

The bottom line is this: What you put in is what you get out. My friend Heidi, who often travels overseas in her work with Food for the Hungry, put it like this: "I realize that as far as my health goes, each day I am making a choice on how I choose to serve God both now and in the future. I can make choices today that will lead me to be an eighty-year-old in a wheelchair, sharing the love of the Lord, or I can choose to live a health-filled life that will allow me to still be out in the mission field, doing what I love and living out how God created me—reaching the unreachable in the darkest places and teaching others about God's heart for the poor." If she doesn't care for her physical well-being, she knows there will be a price to pay in her spiritual, mental, emotional, and social relationships.

Unfortunately, many of us have gotten used to being *underfed* in our quest for spiritual truth and *overfed* in our quest to satisfy physical hunger. We are slowly spiraling further and further into darkness, lies, and bondage. While God has given us everything for our enjoyment, we need to be wise in our choices—including what we eat and drink. When it comes to our physical bodies—bones, hearts, lungs, and brains—it is of utmost importance that we figure out what fuels us best to love.

FOOD: OUR FUEL

In the Eucharist, we drink the juice or wine and eat the bread to remember Christ. Isn't it interesting that God chose food and drink as a way of honoring Him? Why not a specific prayer? Why not a fast? Why not make it a grueling activity like hiking up a mountain while carrying a large hundred-pound rock?

Of course, an act like this would have made a fitness-minded person like me very pleased. But no, I think God chose food and drink because they are the physically sustaining elements of life. If He is the Way, the Truth, and the Life, then He is our spiritually sustaining element of life. The food we choose to eat is another way to honor the God who loved us first. Not in a prideful "Look what I do for God" kind of way, but in an "All I need is You, Lord" way, from a humble and grateful heart.

While many fad diets promote ever-changing direction on how to eat, the Wellness Revelation is not about restricting you by telling you specifically what or how much to eat. *The key is this*: I will ask you to stay constantly conscious of what food does for you and how it makes you feel. The types of food we eat definitely affect how we feel and, in turn, how we do our work. They give us either sustaining fuel (high octane) or draining fuel (low octane).

When we choose wisely, the food we consume will reflect our call to live into Christ's highest purposes for us.

HIGH-OCTANE FUEL VERSUS LOW-OCTANE FUEL

Let's get down to some of the nuts and bolts of a healthy lifestyle—one guided by quality nourishment for our bodies and souls. All food, of course, is broken down into fuel for the body. This fuel is called *glucose* (a fancy word for *sugar*), and it is our bodies' primary energy source and the most readily available form of energy. At the cellular level, glucose is used to keep all the bigger systems of our bodies running smoothly. Just as a car won't run unless there is gasoline in the tank, our bodies can't function without glucose.

This major source of energy is found mostly in a macronutrient called carbo-hydrates. As much as we accuse them of being the bad guys today, we need car-bohydrates. When we don't have them, we know it pretty quickly. For instance, certain parts of our brains derive almost all of their energy from carbohydrates. If you have ever gone on a low-carbohydrate diet, you may have quickly noticed your loss of energy and focus, mentally as well as physically. You may have felt light-headed, dizzy, and lethargic and assumed it was from lack of food. It was actually more likely due to the lack of glucose.

When it comes to getting the glucose we need from our diets, there are poor, good, better, and best fuel choices. Most people think of bread, pasta, or bagels when they hear the word *carbohydrates*, but they are also found in the form of fruits and vegetables.

God was specific with Adam and Eve when He told them what foods they were to eat. "I give you every seed-bearing plant on the face of the whole earth and every tree that has fruit with seed in it. They will be yours for food" (Genesis 1:29). Fruits and vegetables. These are the original foods the Creator designed to be our fuel, prior to the Fall. I think it is quite interesting to realize that before the serpent so cunningly deceived us, we were created to be vegetarians. No animal meat was given for our existence before we fell. But more important, there was no mention of cake, doughnuts, cookies, or the syrupy, sugary liquid we call *soda* either.

This week we are going to expose the poor fuel substitutes. Think of them as cheap, low-octane fuel sources. Sure, they have some "go" power to them, but since they lack purity and cleanliness, using them comes at the risk of our engines eventually blowing up from all the crud and muck they leave behind.

This type of fuel has been manhandled. These foods were created from once-upon-a-time God-given foods, only to be stripped of some if not all of their original nutrients. Most were then beefed up with processed chemicals, all to prolong their shelf life or to produce a bigger flavor explosion so you will keep buying them. Nature has a hard time competing with the party these processed foods create in your mouth!

A few big frauds are white table sugar, high-fructose corn syrup, and enriched white flour. All are carbohydrates, and most of them are found in the boxes, bottles, and bags lining our grocery store shelves. These low-octane, cheap fuel substitutes that hide out in our foods are really just frauds. And if we are not wise, they can steal, kill, and destroy the good design of our bodies.

LOW-OCTANE FUEL

Fraud #1: White Sugar

White sugar is a form of carbohydrate. At one point, it fell from God's design. Sugar actually comes from the root of a beet or a cane, which are both plants. It is first stripped off the sugarcane or sugar beet to become brown sugar. It is then stripped down even more to become basic white table sugar (sucrose). Sucrose is highly addictive and, depending on how much of it you consume, can cause weight gain.

Sucrose is a form of empty calories since the sugar beet or sugarcane loses all its valuable plant nutrients during processing. Your body has no specific use for white sugar; it simply provides an immediate blood sugar surge. When you eat white sugar, your body's metabolic system lights up (which leads to the quick initial high). In order to control the blood sugar spikes, your insulin (a hormone that regulates blood sugar) spikes as well. Sucrose is very beneficial for controlling the plummeting blood sugar levels of someone having a diabetic attack—but too much sucrose can just as easily cause a diabetic attack. Here we see the concept of "permissible but not always beneficial" (see 1 Corinthians 6:12).

Raised insulin levels due to sucrose consumption can cause you to overeat. Shortly after eating sugar-laced foods, you may be just as hungry as you were before. You may also feel your energy plunging, which may lead you to go for the quick fix again. Why does this happen? When you eat white sugar, it raises your level of serotonin, a neurotransmitter that affects your mood. Serotonin is a happy hormone. You feel good upon its release. Yet within an hour of eating sugar, your mood is likely to come crashing down along with your energy. To compensate, your body wants more sugar. You're now in a vicious cycle. An even bigger problem is this: The more sugar you eat, the more resistant your serotonin levels become to sugar, so you need more and more sugar to elevate your mood, causing you to fill up on unnecessary calories with no benefit to the body.

You need to be very aware of the rattling chains of addiction as you wander around in search of more sugar. Sugar is addictive and has the power to fog your thinking. A clear, alert, and conscious mind is crucial as you pursue better health and well-being through a biblical, holistic lifestyle.

Fraud #2: High-Fructose Corn Syrup

Through the 1950s, sucrose (white table sugar) was the number one form of sugar used in the processing and manufacturing of foods. But then food chemists figured out that sucrose can be broken down even further into fructose and glucose (remember glucose is what our bodies are designed to break food into). This led to the creation of the sweet golden liquid called high-fructose corn syrup (HFCS).

HFCS became highly desirable by food manufacturers since it is easier to distribute and has a longer shelf life than sucrose. It also tastes sweeter, meaning a little goes a long way, and it is easier to mix and blend. Almost all boxed foods, from cookies to crackers, contain HFCS.

High-fructose corn syrup is much like table sugar in that it hinders our bodies' ability to regulate weight by making our insulin and blood sugar levels continually oscillate. It is even more stripped down than white table sugar, meaning that it once again interferes with the body's ability to process its own food.

Fraud #3: Enriched White Flour

The definition of *enrich* is "to make rich . . . by the addition or increase of some desirable quality, attribute, or ingredient."[7] Sounds good. Why wouldn't we all want to be enriched? I would like to believe that the Wellness Revelation will enrich you, increasing your quality and quantity of life!

WHEN IT COMES TO OUR PHYSICAL BODIES—BONES, HEARTS, LUNGS, AND BRAINS—IT IS OF UTMOST IMPORTANCE THAT WE FIGURE OUT WHAT FUELS US BEST TO LOVE.

The enriching of foods actually came from good motives. Once upon a time, humans lived through countless famines. Whether the shortages were due to regional weather conditions, lack of resources, or financial destitution, people had to do all that they could to avoid malnourishment or death.

In order to better prepare households for times of famine, the processes of canning and preserving were developed. As a result, foods didn't spoil and were available year-round. Food-processing techniques continued to develop during the twentieth century, providing consumers with more and more prepared foods with longer shelf lives. The downside of food processing is the loss of nutritional value and the addition of preservatives to keep foods from spoiling. This is good for combating famines but bad for overall nutritional value. During the age of famines, the good outweighed the bad, and food processing was a blessing. But famines are unheard of in America today.

Like sugar, enriched flour is very common in processed food. When I was a kid, I loved a peanut butter and jelly sandwich or a grilled cheese made with slices of white Rainbo bread. After school, you could find me in front of the TV watching *The Brady Bunch* while nibbling away on a piece of Rainbo bread, challenging my brother to see who could eat their piece into an animal shape first. You might wonder how something that tastes so good could be so bad.

When manufacturers strip grain of its outside layers, they also remove most of the grain's nutrients. Yet this processed grain has a longer shelf life than whole grain (which means more money and less loss for the food industry), and foods made with this flour have a smoother and softer consistency.

By food industry standards, *enrich* means to put back some of what was taken away, including some of the vitamins that were lost during processing. Whenever you see the term *enriched* on a food label, know that the food is a lower-grade fuel. Some of the original nutrients have been placed back in it, but it has nowhere near the nutritional value it had in its whole state. Enriched flour will give you some energy, but because it's a lower-octane fuel, your gas tank will empty quickly.

Fraud #4: Alcohol

I debated whether or not to talk about alcohol because it is neither a nutrient nor a necessary part of a healthy diet. Yet since more and more people consume alcohol, I think it's worth discussing.

Jesus' first miracle was turning water into wine, and perhaps you, like some others who love Him, enjoy a good glass of wine. However, remember that God's heart for all His kids is that they be free of anything that might take them captive (see Isaiah 61:1). As this week's Bible verse says, "'Everything is permissible for me'—but not everything is beneficial. 'Everything is permissible for me'—but I will not be mastered by anything" (1 Corinthians 6:12). If Paul had been talking about alcohol, I think he would have said: "Listen! You may have a glass of wine, but a glass of wine is never to have you."

If the thought of not being able to have your glass of wine at night makes you panic or break out in a cold sweat, then I would argue that God may be putting His finger on something that is destroying your freedom. Alcohol has you. An idol is present, and God is ready to fight for you. All you need to do is move in step with His powerful Spirit. He loves you too much to not bring this to your attention.

Now let's consider the body's physical response to alcohol. Though alcohol is not a food group, it carries calories. A gram of alcohol has almost twice as many calories as a gram of protein or carbohydrates. It's calorie dense (high calorie count per gram) and calorie dumb (no calorie worth). And when it comes to weight loss, alcohol can be a roadblock. With the first sip, the body recognizes the properties of alcohol and puts it immediately to work as energy to be burned.

While alcohol is in the bloodstream, proteins, carbohydrates, and fats get pushed into the locker room, waiting their turn to run onto the field and be burned for energy. These unused metabolic superstars get sent off into the body to be stored as fat—to be called upon the next time there is a real need for a slow, steady burn. And since alcohol itself has no redeeming nutrients, it clogs up the metabolism until it is used by the body's system.

HIGH-OCTANE FUEL

We need to center our lives more on energy-sustaining foods than on energy-depleting ones. These high-octane foods should be the foundation of our diet. They will not *deplete* us of energy but will *nourish* our bodies from the inside out, transforming the way we think, act, feel, and, yes, even look! Remember, there is power in our food. What besides food can get into the smallest cells in our bodies and change them? From the moment it hits our saliva, which begins breaking it down into various enzymes, food will change who we are for the better or for the worse.

Only God's Holy Spirit and Jesus, the Word, can go that deep, which is one reason He is referred to as "the Bread of Life." The Word has nourishing power and qualities. And so should our "daily bread."

Whole Grains

I give you every seed-bearing plant on the face of the *whole* earth and every tree that has fruit with seed in it. They will be yours for food.
GENESIS 1:29, EMPHASIS MINE

In contrast to the white bread made of enriched flour, whole grains are as close to their natural state as possible and have higher amounts of the vitamins and minerals that our bodies so desperately need. At one point, enriched flour was a whole grain that came from a seed-bearing plant (i.e., wheat). For the sake of big business, it was refined and processed, which robbed it of most of its beneficial qualities as a food source.

Most whole grains are a little nutty in flavor and texture. If you haven't been eating whole grains, they might take some getting used to. We are in the process of retraining our taste buds, so expect a little resistance at first. To this point, if your diet has been composed of low-octane fuel, you have actually been spoon-feeding your taste buds and digestive system. It has all been broken down for you. It is normal to have some challenges, physically, physiologically, and psychologically, when making a shift to the more mature food that God designed for your system.

Be sure to read the ingredient list when you are looking for whole-grain food. The food industry might put "whole" on an item's packaging, but the ingredient label may say "enriched whole wheat flour."

A great way to see if a whole-grain food is really nutritious is to see how many grams of fiber per serving it contains. A quality whole grain will provide you with at least three grams of fiber per serving. Fiber is a key reason why a whole grain is better than an enriched one.

Fiber is a secret weapon for good health and weight management. It functions as a binding agent with fatty acids to prolong the amount of time it takes to empty your stomach. When you eat fiber-rich foods, insulin levels tend to rise at a much slower pace, since sugar is released and absorbed more slowly. You feel full sooner and stay that way longer.

Fiber is also used in cleaning out the body's waste. Without getting graphic, it is best to think of fiber as your body's own pipe-cleaning service. Fiber keeps us from being clogged with crud. As fiber is digested, it cleans out the walls of the large and small intestines, keeping your digestive tract in proper health.

Fiber is always present in healthy foods, so it is no surprise that it is found in just about "every seed-bearing plant . . . and every tree that has fruit with seed in it" (Genesis 1:29).

Fruits and Vegetables

Do you remember that fruits and vegetables are carbohydrates? We tend to think of carbohydrates only as those things that are starchy and bread-like. Yet God created fruits and vegetables to be our main source of fuel.

The Centers for Disease Control and Prevention (CDC) recommends that the average person eat at least three cups of vegetables and two cups of fruit each day. A 2013 study concluded that only about 13 percent of adults in the United States were eating the recommended daily servings of vegetables and about 24 percent were eating the recommended amount of fruit each day.[8] These numbers are not surprising when you consider that 70 percent of Americans currently struggle with their weight.

If you haven't been eating enough fruits and vegetables, *now* is the time to begin. However, if your diet is currently low in dietary fiber, don't raise your fiber intake too quickly, as this may trigger flatulence, bloating, and other undesirable side effects. Your body is going to need time to adjust to mature food. Start by including one or two high-fiber foods daily. Then, every three or four days, add another high-fiber food. Before you know it, your body will begin performing at a whole new level of energy and well-being! The quality of life you enjoy is determined by the quality of foods you eat.

Protein

Getting adequate protein is a necessary element of healthy living. Proteins are the foundation of your structural and functional makeup. Structurally, proteins form most of the solid material in the human body. For example, keratin and collagen are the main building blocks of your muscles, tendons, hair, and skin. Functionally, proteins assist in the activities and processes of the human body. Take hemoglobin, a functional protein that is found in the red blood cells and helps to carry oxygen to all parts of the body. Myosin is a protein in muscle tissue that helps in the contraction of any given muscle. Insulin is a functional protein that helps regulate the storage of glucose—the breakdown of sugar—in the body. Enzymes are proteins that help the productivity of specific chemical reactions in the body. Without protein, we would literally begin to fall apart.

As I've said, I believe we were originally intended to live well and thrive solely on fruits and vegetables (see Genesis 1:29-30), but humans didn't trust God's plan and gave in to the temptation that led to sin. To cover the shame of the naked man and woman, the Lord killed an animal and created the first articles of clothing. I don't have proof, but based on the fact that with the Fall came pain, toil, suffering, and ultimately death (see Genesis 3:16-19), I wonder whether the physical body—biologically, chemically, hormonally, and internally—began to function imperfectly as well, to the point that the basic "building blocks" of muscle (amino acids) began to deconstruct. Is it possible that God killed that animal not only to clothe Adam and Eve but eventually to provide another avenue, beyond fruits and vegetables, for us to rebuild our bodies (see Genesis 9:3)? Maybe. While it *is* possible to get all your protein from a diet of fruits and vegetables alone, it can be challenging to do so in an imperfect world. Therefore, perhaps animal meat is God's provision for those who choose to eat it.

Not all proteins are created equal. The leaner the better, and the cleaner the better. *Lean* means "with fewer naturally occurring fats." *Clean* means "devoid of hormones, additives, and preservatives."

Because consumers seemed to like more fat in their meat, the meat industry began using selective breeding, overfeeding, and the addition of hormones to make animals grow bigger and fatter. We are now beginning to see the negative effects of these actions. When children eat meat with added steroids and growth hormones, their overall growth is affected. Eating meat containing these additives has also led to an earlier onset of menstruation in girls, putting them at a slightly higher risk for breast cancer and other chronic diseases. Finally, antibiotics administered to animals for rapid growth can expose humans to drug-resistant bacteria. To avoid these effects, be sure to read labels carefully when purchasing animal protein.

Dairy, an animal by-product, can be a good source of protein. However, it is an inflammatory food for many people. In fact, it's estimated that 75 percent of the world's population has a hard time digesting dairy. Physical challenges like sinus infections, eczema, and irritable bowel syndrome can be connected to a person's inability to properly digest dairy. Symptoms like bloating, flatulence, diarrhea, and constipation are common side effects of being lactose intolerant. Fortunately, a diet filled with fruits and vegetables—particularly leafy greens—will cover your calcium and basic vitamin and mineral needs.

Fats: Not All Are Created Equal

When did *fat* become such a bad word? Before I talk about fat, a necessary macronutrient in food, I would like to talk about fat, the necessary grace that is found in our bodies. Fat is a part of God's glorious and good design, and nobody on planet Earth could survive without some fat on their frame. If having fat makes us fat, then we are all *fat*!

Fats are not the absolute evil they are often made out to be. They are a necessary part of a healthy diet. They play a vital role in maintaining healthy skin and hair, insulating body organs against shock, regulating body temperature, and promoting healthy cell function. They also serve as energy stores for the body. Fat is a major source of energy and aids in the absorption of vitamins A, D, E, and K. Both animal-derived and plant-derived food products contain fat. When eaten in moderation, fats aid in proper growth, development, and maintenance of good health, particularly those found in God-created foods such as nuts, seeds, fruits, vegetables, and legumes. Now before you run off to the corner doughnut store, consider the very real differences between good and bad fats.

Good fats: polyunsaturated/monounsaturated. Polyunsaturated and mono-unsaturated fats may help lower your blood cholesterol levels. They are found in plant oils like olive oil, peanut oil, sunflower oil, and sesame oil. These oils come from vegetables and seeds that are pressed (preferably cold pressed since heat can destroy many of their beneficial enzymes). Other sources of good fats include avocados, peanut butter, and various nuts and seeds.

Not-so-good fats: hydrogenated oils/saturated fats/trans fats. Hydrogenated oils of any kind are not part of God's plan for healthy eating. The hydrogenation process turns liquid vegetable oil into solid fat. The goal of partial hydrogenation is to add hydrogen atoms to unsaturated fats to make them more saturated. These kinds of saturated fats have a higher melting point, making them very attractive for baking and extending the shelf life of baked goods.

Partially hydrogenated oils contain trans fat, which should be avoided. They lower your good cholesterol and raise your bad cholesterol, thereby increasing your risk for heart disease. That is why we see manufacturers touting their products as "zero trans fats."

Be sure to read your labels. Your best bet is to be sure that your food is free from partially (or fully) hydrogenated oils.

As you compare your options, remember that not all saturated fats are created equal—just as not all foods are created equal. The operative word here is *created*—food closest to its original source with minimal to no manufacturing or processing involved is best for your body. For example, coconut oil is a naturally occurring saturated fat that many believe is an exception to the "don't eat saturated fat" rule. Unlike other saturated fats and trans fats, coconut oil can help establish healthy cholesterol levels.

In fact, what is true about fats is true of all food types: The closer a food is to its original design—free from artificial enhancers or machine processing—the better it is for you.

RESPOND

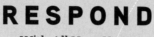

With All Your Heart

> Now that you have completed some simple health assessments, you can begin to move forward. But before you do so, I would like to help you lay a healthy foundation from which to start. This week's videos will help you train your core strength and stability, as well as your mobility. They will also talk about healthy posture and alignment. If you have struggled with excessive pain in your body before or after a workout, this week is truly going to help. Before we move more, let's move better! You can access the Wellness Revelation Workout Calendar on page 240.

THE EATING PLAN

The Detox Fast

Last week you were invited to participate in a standard fast: to get spiritually hungry for more of God by giving up the physical comfort of food for a period of time. This week, we will focus on retraining our taste buds. I would like to ask you to prayerfully consider taking a rest not from all food but from certain kinds of foods—white sugar, enriched flour, high-fructose corn syrup, and/or alcohol. You do not have to remove these all at once. Try to choose the one(s) that God is calling to your attention now. God never despises small steps.

If you remove this low-octane fuel from your life and replace it with high-octane fuel, I can promise that you will have more clarity and energy than you have had in a long time. You will also achieve weight loss at a consistent and natural pace.

This is an element fast, which removes from your diet those foods that may have mastered you. Whatever you decide to fast from, let me encourage you to be all in! A lukewarm element fast will be filled with tedious temptation and "chasing after the wind" (Ecclesiastes 1:14). You will need to pray when you are faced with temptation. You will most likely find yourself praying a lot to loosen the bonds of your cravings. Be sure to call out for mercy and stay connected to the Vine because apart from Him you can do nothing (see John 15:5). Don't forget: God loves a fast that is done with the right heart—one that wants to be transformed, obedient to the will of God.

Remember the reason you agreed to join the Wellness Revelation program: You desire to live a healthy and whole life so you are freed up to love yourself (in a healthy and righteous way) and to love others. This is an active and sacrificial process. You are the living sacrifice (see Romans 12:1). Always stay honest with God and surrender your strength to Him. Never doubt His greatness within you. He is stronger than any craving.

While you are detox fasting, eating will feel somewhat unfamiliar. You will experience some body rebellion, such as headaches, hunger, and cravings. Don't panic. Keep your peace. A life lived according to the flesh doesn't like newness unless it's connected to more pleasure. The flesh is all about comfort, which it often seeks through pleasures of the flesh. However, your body is designed for homeostasis (equilibrium), making the various functions of the body inter-dependent on one another. When you give in to unhealthy pleasures of the flesh, the peaceful interplay of your body's working systems breaks down.

Your body, soul, and spirit were created to work together. Before now, your soul (the seat of your appetites, dreams, and desires) and your body (the frame with the ability to execute these desires) have been running the show. They are used to getting what they want while your spirit (your desire to know God, love Him, and worship Him) has been accused of being insignificant and weak and forced by your flesh to sit down and shut up. But now, as we use this fast as a tool, your spirit is being asked to stand up and take its rightful place as the leader of the pack.

Phase One: Entering the Cocoon

When my kids were small, one of their favorite books was *The Very Hungry Caterpillar*, the story of a caterpillar doing what caterpillars do—eating good, naturally occurring foods like blueberries, strawberries, oranges, and plums. But the caterpillar is not satisfied with those foods. He stumbles upon and eats "chocolate cake, one ice-cream cone, one pickle, one slice of Swiss cheese, one slice of salami, one lollipop, one piece of cherry pie, one sausage, one cupcake, and one slice of watermelon."[9] Sound familiar? He'd gotten distracted, but he still had a chance to turn things around. This very fat caterpillar now built himself a cocoon.

We need cocoons occasionally. We need times to visit the dark places and do what is hard so that new and beautiful things can emerge. We never go into a cocoon alone, because we always go with God. In our rush to see and experience beauty, we often try to avoid struggle and suffering. But just as the caterpillar had to die to his old self and existence in order for his new life as a butterfly to begin, so must we. The time in the cocoon will be trying, but out of the trial will come true beauty.

For at least the next three days, I ask you to enter your own personal "cocoon" and fast from the element(s) you know God is putting His finger on. For some of you, the thought of going three days without [fill in the blank] makes your feet sweat and your stomach feel sick! You are on the right path to greater holiness and wholeness when you know you will need the Comforter to comfort you. Seek God's heart when you long to give up and reach for your go-to comfort food. Remember that if you seek God with all your heart, you will find Him (see Jeremiah 29:13). And you may even find that God will give you the grace to go longer than three days—maybe even three weeks or three months. Who knows? The whole point is to become utterly dependent on the voice of Love to lead you and give you strength. You call, and He will answer.

Food Suggestions List

PROTEIN (portion aware)
**Baked beans (canned; be
  sugar aware)**
Bison
Black-eyed peas
Canadian bacon
Chicken breast
Chickpeas
Eggs
**Ground beef (lean,
  10–20 percent fat)**
Ground turkey
Lamb
Lean beef
**Lean deli ham
  (hormone-free)**
Lentils
Lima beans
Navy beans
Peas
Pinto beans
Pork
Sashimi
Seafood
Smoked salmon
Soybeans
Tofu
Turkey bacon
Turkey breast
Veal

DAIRY (portion aware)
Greek yogurt—unflavored
Milk substitutes (nut, rice,
  coconut)

FRUITS (great snacks)
Apples
Apricots
Bananas
Blackberries
Blueberries
Cherries
Grapefruit
Grapes
Kiwis
Lemons/limes
Mangoes
Oranges
Papayas
Peaches
Pears
Pineapples
Plums
Raspberries
Strawberries
All other fruits

BREAD/GRAIN
(portion aware)
Barley
**Bran/high-fiber
  cereal**
Brown basmati rice
Buckwheat
Bulgur
Kavli thin crackers
Muesli cereal
**Oatmeal (old fashioned/
  steel cut)**
Quinoa

Sprouted breads
  (e.g. Ezekiel)
**Whole-grain high-fiber
  bread**
*Whole-grain high-fiber
  tortillas*
Whole-grain pita bread

VEGETABLES
Artichokes
Asparagus
Avocados
Beans
Beets
Bell peppers (all colors)
Broccoli
Brussels sprouts
Cabbage
Carrots
Cauliflower
Celery
Collard greens
Corn
Cucumbers
Edamame
Eggplant
Kale
Leeks
Lettuce (all leafy greens)
Mushrooms
Okra
Olives
Onions
Peppers, hot
Pickles

Potatoes (portion aware)
Pumpkin
Radishes
Snow peas
Spinach
Squash
Sweet potatoes
  (portion aware)
Tomatoes
Yams (portion aware)
Zucchini
All other vegetables

CONDIMENTS
Garlic
Herbs/spices
Hummus
Mayonnaise (portion aware)
Mustard
Parmesan cheese
Raw honey (portion aware)
Salsa
Soy sauce, low sodium
Sriracha sauce
Stevia

Tabasco
Teriyaki sauce
  (sugar aware)
Vinegar (white,
  apple cider)
Worcestershire sauce

FATS/OILS (portion aware)
Almond butter—no added
  ingredients
Canola oil
Coconut oil
Corn oil
Flaxseed/flaxseed oil
Hazelnuts
Macadamia nuts
Mayonnaise
Natural nut butter (peanut,
  almond, cashew, etc.)—
  no added ingredients
Olive oil
Peanut oil
Salad dressing
  (sugar aware)
Sesame oil

Sunflower oil
Vegetable oil
Vegetable oil sprays
All other nuts

BEVERAGES
Water (filtered if needed)
Decaffeinated coffee
Decaffeinated tea

FASTING
High-fructose corn syrup/
  fructose
Hydrogenated/partially
  hydrogenated oils
Refined sugar (cookies,
  pastries, ice cream, frozen
  yogurt, etc.)
White enriched flour
Artificial sweeteners
  (the novel sweetener stevia
  is an exception; enjoy
  modestly)
Alcohol

Remember: These are suggestions, not prescriptions. Please prayerfully submit the items and ideas listed here to the Lord, seeking His will for you in this time and in concert with the *whole* work He wants to do for and in you.

For some of you, this will be a call to greater self-control—for others it will be a call to looser self-regulation. He's got your answer.

If you have special dietary needs or concerns, please consult your health practitioner of choice.

In my distress I called to the LORD;
    I cried to my God for help.
From his temple he heard my voice;
    my cry came before him, into his ears.

PSALM 18:6

Come to me, all who labor and are heavy laden, and I will give you rest.

MATTHEW 11:28, ESV

Studies show that on average it takes around three weeks to break an old craving or habit and to start a new one. It takes up to three months before that new habit becomes established as a part of your daily life. God loves it when we follow Him into situations where we are totally dependent on Him.

For at least three days, with the God-supported hope of going three weeks, choose one or more elements that you sense the Lord is asking you to take a rest from in your daily diet:

A rest from sugar or anything sweet
A rest from hydrogenated oils and enriched flour (foods that are found
    in boxes or processed and passed through a window)
A rest from alcohol

Ask God when He is asking you to begin, and I am confident He will also tell you when to end your fast. Don't panic when your body throws a tantrum in all its various forms—headaches, irritability, and anxiety. That's exactly the time when things are getting good and you are closing in on some newfound freedom. Stay armored in His Word and in your cocoon until God says it's the right time to come out. He knows you want freedom. And He wants your freedom even more than you do. Trust Him within your ugly, inner-child, tantrum moments. He's not offended by them.

How to Eat While Cocooning

The Food Suggestions List on pages 76–77 is filled with a selection of high-octane fuel choices. I hope this gives you a jump start on the items you can stock in your cabinets as well as foods to look for when eating out. Keep in mind, vegetables and fruits are your very best friends. If a food is not on the list but grew out of the ground, by all means take a bite and enjoy it to the glory of God! *Disclaimer*: No one food plan can heal and meet the needs of all people, but eating whole, high-octane, minimally manhandled food is always a great place to start!

I would like to introduce you to a simple and sound way of nourishing your body; it's what I call the "4S" of feeding your body and soul.

1. *Slow.* Oh no. Now I've done it. I am asking you to slow down in a world that says, "Go faster! Do more! Be more!" Think of your slowing down to eat as a rebellious, joyful act of celebration. Slowing down in today's culture is *counter*cultural. It's also the only hope you have for letting God have the right of way—for letting Him lead. He wants to fight this battle for you, but you will need to be still *before* your enemies as you move in a new direction (see Exodus 14:14).

   Practice taking a moment to breathe and give thanks to God for what you are about to eat. Do this not as a robotic ritual but as a way to invite God in, to let Him sit at the head of your table and eat with you. Thank Him for making good on His promises to give you all you need so that you do not have to worry (see Matthew 6:31-33). Just take a moment to be grateful. I can promise you . . . a grateful heart is a full heart. It never wants for more.

2. *Sufficient.* If you classify yourself as an overeater, one of your challenges is not just what to eat but how much to put on your plate. The key word here is *plate*. Though I am not into scales and measurements, I encourage you

to purchase some eight-inch plates if you don't already have them. Over the years, our increasing appetites have led to bigger and bigger plates, causing us to eat more than we need. Make it a habit to eat from a real plate. The act of "plating" a meal (even if it's just a sandwich and some veggie sticks) is an act of honoring God—the One who gives you food—as well as yourself as you take time to sit down, rest, refresh, and refuel.

So what should you put on your eight-inch plate? First divide it into thirds.

Fill one-third of your plate with a serving of lean, clean protein.

Fill one-third of your plate with a serving of a whole-grain carbohydrate.

Fill one-third of your plate with fruits and/or vegetables.

If you notice your body does better with less grain, then taper back for a meal or two. The same thing applies to meat. Supplement all of the above with a serving of "good fat" as desired (e.g., coconut oil to cook your eggs in; peanut butter on your toast; a side of avocado).

If you have difficulty determining serving sizes, feel free to pull out some measuring cups and spoons to get in touch with reality. But don't plan on hanging those suckers around your neck or carrying them in your purse. After a few days of reality checking, you and your sound, renewed mind will have a good idea of what a healthy portion size is. Here are some good guidelines:

Meats: A four-ounce serving is about the size of a deck of cards or the palm of your hand.

Whole grains: One cup is the size of your fist.

Vegetables: Two cups of raw, leafy vegetables is the size of two open hands.

Cooked vegetables: One cup equals one fist.

Fruit: One-half cup is about what fits in the cup of your palm.

Not all serving sizes are treated equally. For example, one average-sized apple is considered a serving. Though it won't necessarily fit in the palm of your hand, it can rest in there. Use your best judgment. And remember that it's nearly impossible to eat too many fruits and vegetables.

3. *Satisfied.* You may need to ask the Lord to awaken your sense of hunger and fullness. If you have used food over the years to feed the slightest pangs of hunger, your brain may have lost its ability to tell you when you are full. Praise God that He is the restorer of all things. Whatever the locusts ate, He will return (see Joel 2:25). As you slow down while eating, invite your good Father to tell you when you have had enough. *Countless* people have told me that God awakened their sense of fullness just because they asked. So go ahead . . . ask.

   Use the Hunger Scale in your Moving Forward Journal. Remember that it is based on a scale of 1 to 5—1 being ravenously hungry and 5 being stuffed and needing to loosen your pants. Do your part to keep your hunger and satisfaction between a 2 and a 4 throughout your day. This is where eating steadily makes a difference.

   Pay attention to your hunger. If you are finding you are still *very* hungry after eating a meal with a well-balanced plate of high-octane food for fuel, then you might be restricting your food too much out of fear. Eating too many quality calories is rare, especially for those with weary and confused hearts who have battled weight their whole lives. Be free . . . be satisfied, and be not stuffed. Ask God for the grace to know the difference.

4. *Steady.* Make it a holy goal (to the best of your ability) to keep your blood sugar level. Radical spikes and plummets of blood sugar can be behind some of your most unpleasant binges.

Eat three meals a day with a snack in between as needed. This may seem like a lot of eating at first. If that's the case, it's likely that your metabolism has been suppressed by years of bingeing, restricting, and maybe even purging. Eating more steadily throughout the day is like throwing a log on a fire that you want to burn continually. By consistently feeding the fire of your metabolism with good and steady fuel, you will cleanse your body, soul, and mind from the gunk and leftover buildup that come from ravenous bingeing. Ask God to gently but firmly help you increase your desire to eat a little more steadily throughout the day.

If moments of high hunger or low energy occur, try eating every two to three hours by incorporating two snacks a day: one after breakfast and one after lunch. The snack can be as simple as a handful of nuts and some dried fruit. (Snacks don't require a plate, but please don't let me stop you from slowing down. I have been known to enjoy an apple and a peanut butter packet in my car, in a moment of silence.)

Make a conscious effort not to go to bed on a full stomach. Try to finish up your nourishment for the day within two to three hours of bedtime. Remember, there's a reason the first meal of the day is called *breakfast*. We eat to "break the fast" that started before we went to bed—not when we went to bed. With that being said, don't push your bedtime back so you can stay up longer to eat. (I know how our crazy minds work.)

For God has not given us a spirit of fear, but of power and of love and of a sound mind.

2 TIMOTHY 1:7, NKJV

Phase Two: Coming Out of the Cocoon

If you do the full three weeks in your cocoon, complete weeks 4 and 5 in this book as you continue to fast from your chosen foods. In week 6, we will discuss the process of coming out of your cocoon.

If you come out sooner than three weeks, begin by celebrating God's goodness, and do not feel shame that you didn't get as far as three weeks. That shame game we play is part of what steals the health and wholeness that are ours as sons and daughters of God. If you are wondering what eating looks like now, turn to week 6, where "The Butterfly—Freedom" phase is covered in depth. Even if you have come out of your cocoon, be sure to continue working through weeks 4 and 5 in this book.

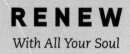

RENEW

With All Your Soul

Set aside some disciplined and focused time this week to read, study, pray, and apply God's Word to your life.

1. Our lives can easily become too self-centered. Read Colossians 1:15-18. If we take this passage to heart, how will it correct our perspective? In what ways do you ensure that God is leading and directing your life?

2. Looking back, can you remember a time when you clearly desired something other than God's purpose for you? What happened?

3. Read John 5:30. Does this describe you right now? Are what you do and how you live purposefully aimed at pleasing God or pleasing yourself? What do you need to do to change your purpose to more closely line up with His purpose for you? Be as specific as possible.

4. If you believe you have been purposeful in pleasing God, what has happened in your life that has gotten you off track with your weight or health?

5. According to Genesis 1:28, our purpose is to "be fruitful and increase in number." Beyond procreation, this means we are to produce what is good. Does this describe your life? Why or why not?

6. Frederick Buechner said, "The vocation for you is the one in which your deep gladness and the world's deep need meet."[10] I believe that God has given each one of us an individual talent, gift, voice, vocation, passion, and desire for whatever brings us the greatest joy and can add value to His Kingdom. What gifts has God given to you? How well are you embodying the true peace and joy that comes in living according to the way He designed you?

7. If you are not sure of your purpose, or if you want to be sure that you are living completely in His will for your life, read Matthew 7:7-8. According to this passage, what do you need to do to find your purpose? Be persistent and continue to pray that God will reveal His deeper purpose for your life in Him.

Living Sacrifices for His Purpose

8. We talked about the city of Corinth and how many people there used their bodies in ways that displeased the Lord. Read 1 Corinthians 6:19-20. To whom do our bodies belong?

9. What do you think it means to honor God with our bodies?

10. Just as Christ's body, the church, has many parts, so does your individual body. Your body consists of the physical (heart, lungs, skin, muscle, blood), the mental/emotional (thoughts and feelings), and the spiritual (the qualities that make you *you*; for example, living for His purpose). Each has a job to do that affects the whole. When you are not honoring God with your body (the physical element), how does that affect all other parts of your life— mental/emotional, social, and spiritual—and your ability to live out His purpose? Please address all areas and be specific:

Physical:

Mental/emotional:

Social:

Spiritual:

Father,

Thank You for loving all of me. Now I give You not just my heart but my body too. I want more of You. I know that to make room for You, I need to allow less room for things without eternal value. I believe You care about all the details of my life, including what I put in my body and what I do with my body. Help me to turn to You when I am tempted to fill up on things that do not satisfy. Fill me instead with Your Word so that I may live according to Your good and pleasing will for my life. I desire to be healthy, whole, and free in body, soul, and spirit. Thank You that You want this for me too.
✝ *Amen.*

RELATE

With All Your Mind and Strength

The following questions are designed to help you apply all you've learned this week to your fitness journey. Get with your accountability partner or small group and work honestly through these questions. Consider journaling your answers with God before sharing with your partner or group.

1. What food or foods have been mastering you?

2. If you cannot have the food(s) you want, what happens to your body? How do you feel? Be as specific as possible.

3. Describe a time in your life when food was a comfort to you.

4. Has food been serving you, or have you been serving food? If you have been serving food, what has it stolen from you?

RECIPROCATE

Fit for the Kingdom in Nigeria

**by Kari Jo Shephard,
Revelation Wellness Ambassador**

My family and I have been serving in Jos, Nigeria, for almost six years. My husband is a physician, our three boys attend an international school, and I teach fitness classes twice a week to missionaries and local Nigerians as a certified Revelation Wellness ambassador.

Two of my students are Hanatu, a teacher, and her daughter, Ladi, a high school student. Every Thursday afternoon for the past year, they have faithfully entered a classroom of a different variety—the room where we meet for our Kingdom Fit workouts. In this classroom, they are active and vibrant participants. Not only do they exercise, they enter God's presence through movement, God's Word, and prayer.

One particular Thursday just before class, my mind and heart were not very excited about the prospect of leading a class intended to uplift and encourage people. I had been struggling through a rough week. But out of a sense of obligation I went, and I started class as I always do—by reading Scripture and praying for God to speak to us through our time in movement and worship. I read the day's Scripture, Psalm 30:11, which was the cry of my heart: "You turned my wailing into dancing; you removed my sackcloth and clothed me with joy." After I'd finished, I decided to open up about the week I'd had, explaining that I didn't truly *want* to be there but was trusting God to turn my wailing into dancing and to clothe me with joy. I invited the students to join me in this plea for the Lord to transform our attitudes.

Class went on as normal, and thankfully I sensed joy developing inside me as I continued to move and focus on the Lord. We all worked up quite a sweat before beginning the cooldown.

After class we make cleaning the room a community event. We close windows and curtains, roll up mats, and gather our belongings together. As we were putting everything away, Ladi approached me. Though usually a very quiet and reserved young woman, she began to open up about how she was struggling due to her brother attending university in another country. She told me how much she missed him and that she had been feeling depressed. Since attending Kingdom Fit classes, however, she had been greatly encouraged and was feeling much better about the situation. When Hanatu came over to get her daughter, she also told me how encouraged she had been to hear about my tough week because she had been having a similar experience. She was glad to know she wasn't alone in her struggles.

Heaven came down to earth that day. God knew our hearts and what they needed, and true to form, He did not disappoint us. He met each of us in our need and *turned our wailing into dancing and clothed each of us with His great joy!* Whether students share what God is doing or not, I know He is at work through each class and in every heart. God is in the business of encouraging and drawing all of us into deeper relationship with Him.

REST IN HIS STRENGTH AND SUFFICIENCY

My flesh and my heart may fail, but God is the strength
of my heart and my portion forever.

PSALM 73:26

Are you familiar with the weight-loss game? I think it is fair to say almost all of us are. (If you have never struggled with your weight, consider yourself blessed and pray that you never have to.) It is a frustrating exercise that usually starts the weekend before D-day Monday—the day we swear to ourselves that we are going to buckle down and drop the pounds.

We are strong in spirit—like prizefighters ready to take on the match. Yet isn't it funny that the weekend before the fateful Monday, we find ourselves at our favorite restaurant eating our "last meal"? This action sends a message to our brains that we are about to begrudgingly enter a dark and scary place, a place we wish we didn't have to go. We share our last moments with an old friend and comforter—food. We know that the next day, week, or months will bring challenges and temptations that will make us very uncomfortable.

With that attitude, we are overwhelmed a day or two into the process. We fear that we will fail once again, which leads to feelings of negative self-worth. Or we might fear success. We are afraid of what lost pounds might cost us or the expectations we might place upon ourselves if we reach our goals. There is fear of not getting what we want and fear of getting what we want. Now what? We're stuck. No wonder we quickly surrender and go back to old habits.

Remember, food is not the enemy here. Food is a *good* thing. God created *all* things that are good, and food is one of His glorious creations. Our problem is when our *good* thing becomes our *god* thing. God wants Himself, not food, to be our source of comfort. When we place too much importance on food, whether by controlling and obsessing over it (anorexia, bulimia) or by overconsuming it to feed a need beyond hunger (bingeing), we are using food functionally to save us from our fears.

My question is: Why do we create this "last meal" scene? Why do we suffer such feelings of despair and drudgery when faced with the reality that we need to lose weight or become healthier by changing our relationship with food?

I propose the following: We have underestimated our own strength and, even worse, the strength of God in us. We fear failure and temptation so much that we indulge ourselves in our flesh one last time. We think we are preparing ourselves for entering into battle, but metaphorically speaking, we are hanging our heads and longingly looking back at what *was*. We are like soldiers about to head off to war, who want to spend one more evening in the arms of their loved ones. But while the soldiers choose to spend their final moments with people who can give and receive love, our lover is food—something that can never love us back in a way that calls us out of a dark pit or a kitchen pantry.

I would suggest that in the past, we have entered the weight-loss battle relying on our own strength. We see an infomercial or a social media post, read a new diet book, or find a weight-loss blog and think, *That's it! The time is now! I can do this! I know better, and it's time for me to do better! I don't care what it takes; even if I have to hire a personal trainer to tell me what to do, I will do it! Enough is enough!* We might even put a holy cherry on top by declaring, "And the Bible tells me so!" to seal the deal.

Somehow, though, we overlook the Bible's warning about fighting temptation in our own strength: "If you live according to the flesh you will die, but if by the Spirit you put to death the deeds of the body, you will live" (Romans 8:13, ESV).

We often begin the weight-loss battle in the flesh. We think, *This time I will be strong enough; I will have the ultimate willpower. This time I have a trainer and some accountability. This time I have this awesome new piece of home exercise equipment. This time I have the best diet plan!* We convince ourselves that if we are strong enough, we can do anything, be anything, or have anything.

Jesus warned us that our spirits would be willing but our bodies would be weak (see Mark 14:38). But perhaps the converse could be said as well: that our

---

Remember to use your **Moving Forward Journal** this week to track your food and water intake, as well as to remain focused on this week's Scripture verse. You can download a copy at www.revelationwellness.org/book/workout or photocopy the template on page 239.

bodies may be willing, but our spirits are weak. The point is, no matter what we do or where we go, we all have blind spots—weaknesses in spirit, soul, or body. Rather than letting that discourage us, I propose that perhaps our weak spots are opportunities to see God work—places in us, ordained by Him, that He uses to make Himself known. Sometimes we can feel Him carry us through our struggles; other times we might not feel Him at all. But our feelings don't change the fact that Jesus came as Emmanuel, God with us. And wherever He is, there is abundant strength. As King David exclaimed near the end of his life: "In your hands are strength and power to exalt and give strength to all" (1 Chronicles 29:12).

That's not to say that some people don't lose weight simply by drawing on sheer willpower. I've watched clients who didn't know God or who didn't make the connection between their bodies and spirits achieve their fitness goals. The only card they had to play in the weight-loss game was their own personal power. They made the hard choices and did the hard work. They did their happy dance when they got to wear their size [fill in the blank] jeans. Yet I discovered something interesting: In every case, their happiness was short-lived. Once they lost the weight, one of two scenarios quickly played out:

Weight-loss scenario #1: Led by the flesh, they become so obsessed with the "new them," or being thin, or working out and eating right, that they do it for the wrong reasons. Their mentality is *If a little is good, then more is better.* They are never really satisfied and always look for more (*If I could only lose five more pounds* . . .). Their desire for the perfect weight, size, or look becomes insatiable. Many even develop body dysmorphic disorder, which stems from a warped sense of what they look like and causes them to obsess about perceived flaws in their appearance. They look in the mirror and cannot see truth. Their consistent focus on their flaws amplifies the lies. This deceitful path steals time and energy from God, family, and friends.

People who depend solely on willpower to lose weight run the risk of becoming consumed by their new identity. They may develop a constant need to be at the gym or to further develop their physical beauty. They may be so obsessed by what they can and cannot eat that no one wants to go to lunch with them anymore. The source of their bondage and idolatry shifts from gluttony and neglect to vanity. They are abusing food again, but this time with a more legalistic view.

Before judging those who fall into this track, we need to remember that we are all guilty of exchanging one idol for another. Just as Satan often succeeds at using food as the bait to steal our health and to distract us from living for God, he eagerly awaits on the other side of good health, ready to get us to hyperfocus on our remaining imperfections. Then he tempts us with the lie that we can do better, that there's always more for the taking.

There's nothing wrong with improving our lives. Jesus came to give us more life—to proclaim good news to the captive, to give sight to the blind and healthy legs to the lame, and to make broken hearts whole. He knows that when we ask for a smaller waistline, we are really searching for love and belonging. But like any good father, God reserves the right to get in our way and say, "Enough." His grace is our sufficiency. What more could we possibly need?

Weight-loss scenario #2: Led by the flesh, at some point people drawing only on willpower see their strength fail. "For . . . the weakness of God is stronger than human strength" (1 Corinthians 1:25). As the personal strength meter goes down, they slip up. The "one time" becomes another time and yet another time. This repeats over and over until they have slowly slipped right back into their old habits. They again seek to fill the void with food, work, sex, consumption, or excess. They find comfort in the familiar.

The problem is that until they connect to *the* source—the Spirit, the source of all true power, who is God in them—they will fail. God offers them something much better: "The Spirit God gave us does not make us timid, but gives us power, love and self-discipline" (2 Timothy 1:7). True and lifelong self-discipline based on blessed obedience does not come from ourselves but from God in us by the power of the Holy Spirit. He is our Strength and our Sufficiency.

A few years ago, I had a close-up view of what it looks like when someone draws on God's strength and sufficiency. Each year my team and I train people to hike the Grand Canyon in one day as part of a fund-raising event we call Rim to Him. For us, nothing is worth doing if it's not about finding more of God or giving God more. And what better place to find more of God than inside one of the seven wonders of the world?

That year Tracy, one of our first-time hikers, took me to church—in other words, she preached! Tracy gave words to the battle I felt God was calling me to help people fight—the fight for freedom in their bodies. After half a year of faithful training, Tracy started her hike across the Grand Canyon in high spirits and with even higher hopes. Her enthusiasm was contagious. I noticed that when others came near her, she was encouraging and kind. From the start, she seemed to take her steps with great ease, as if her feet were playing music as she moved down the dusty trail into the depths of the Grand Canyon. Tracy smiled, she was engaging, and she stayed upbeat—until her body hit the proverbial fitness wall. After fifteen hours of hiking up and down the canyon, Tracy was closing in on the final mile of the twenty-four-mile trek. As we watched the sun set over a dimly lit tree line, I saw Tracy fading. Her feet were no longer playing a catchy melody; they were dragging. With her stride shortening and her desire to speak waning, I was concerned. In a quiet moment, when all we could hear was the sound of our feet and our breath and we were surrounded by a few others who needed renewed strength, I asked, "Tracy, how are you feeling? You good?"

My question worked like smelling salts under her nose. On cue, she snapped out of her foot-shuffle trance and said with convincing vim, "Oh, me? I'm doing great! My body is just going to have to catch up!"

What a violent act of hope! In her physical poverty, Tracy made a withdrawal on the Kingdom of God inside her, a Kingdom that has no lack, and she spoke life from her spirit toward her flesh. She told her body not to forget who was in charge. In one powerful statement, she directed her doubts to take their place in the back of the bus and to sit down, shut up, and keep their hands to themselves.

I'm doing great. My body is just going to have to catch up. Those are words that will never leave me when it's time to fight the good fight of faith. We must never put our hope in what we feel. Feelings are meant to be felt, not drive what we do.

NO MORE YO-YO DIETING

In *The Wellness Revelation*, we are striving for more than weight loss. We want a life gained. A life of freedom. A life that gets its power and strength from the Source, where no mountain is too high and no valley is too low. When we have life, we can give life. Below are three attributes necessary for a person who is seeking to live in the freedom Christ offers:

Mindfulness

The choices we make every day have consequences. Jesus promised that "blessed . . . are those who hear the word of God and obey it" (Luke 11:28). If we do as God commands, we have done all we can to avoid negative consequences. This is not to say that bad things won't happen to good people, but even then, we can find peace and purpose when we remain humble and teachable, willing to display God's glory in our suffering while maintaining our faith in His goodness.

Only through mindfulness—living intentionally—can we keep our minds set on things above so we remember that we belong to Christ and are His agents of change here on earth. Living with this mind-set reminds us that every choice we make is important.

When we learn to slow down and stop living on autopilot, we are more aware of the choices we make, the words we say, and the actions we take. We become engaged in and fully present to life. We remember we have God's good favor even in the toughest of circumstances. We develop a mind like Christ and a mind for Christ.

Balance versus Wholeheartedness

Balance. What a tricky and very Zen-like word. I used to think balance was the goal that would lead to a great life. As a young wife, mom, and ministry leader, I wanted to be the woman who had everything humming and working in perfect order. After all, I was a wellness professional; if anyone was supposed to achieve balance, it should be me. Right? Wrong. The more I strove for balance, the more frustrated I became. I felt like a circus performer trying to keep all my plates spinning on a stick while riding a unicycle.

I have come to realize that balance doesn't exist. Balance, as the world defines it, would require me to be a jack-of-all-trades and a master of none. I'd have to devote one piece of myself to being a good wife who made sure the house was clean, dinner was in the oven, and my husband felt loved. Another piece of me would have to clean up after my kids, get them to all their doctor's appointments, and be sure their teachers were happy with their progress. Yet another piece of me would be striving to keep my clients happy and myself in shape and up to date on developments in the fitness world. A final piece of me would try to spend time seeking after God. And let me be honest . . . when I was attempting to keep my life balanced, that last part of me was sometimes the part I would overlook—even though I knew it was the most important. Trying to "balance" my life felt more like relying on excellent management skills than on being fully present and enjoying the good things in life.

Instead of seeking balance, I encourage you to seek wholehearted living, which means showing up to every circumstance completely as you are and where you are, and giving what you can. Wholehearted living means doing everything with great passion and purpose, even when you are asked to do something you are not good at. Still you show up, bringing your unique voice and your kind heart inside your one-of-a-kind beautiful body, believing you have something to offer that will create hope, love, and life in yourself and others. Wholehearted people know who they are and whose they are. They know they can offer value and worth in every situation, even if it's simply by bringing their presence. They give what they can and don't shrink back in fear of being judged. And they don't hold back for fear of running out because they know how to go to God, their source, to get more of what they need. You don't have to be proficient at something to be effective at it. By showing up and being completely themselves, wholehearted people foster peace, joy, and growth in those around them because these qualities flow from within them.

The problem is, we can't give away what we don't have. We won't be wholehearted until we begin to believe and act upon this truth: *God loves me, accepts me, and tells me I am right with Him.* This is called having righteousness, or being aligned with the all-encompassing love of God. It is by faith we are made righteous (see Romans 1:17). To be righteous is to be positioned with God's rightness—His right way of feeling, thinking, speaking, and acting in all circumstances. We must not forget that God is right. He is the Way, the Truth, and the Life (see John 14:6). We think we know the way, but we don't know it unless we humble ourselves and seek God's heart. He holds the map and the

BY SHOWING UP AND BEING COMPLETELY THEMSELVES, WHOLEHEARTED PEOPLE FOSTER PEACE, JOY, AND GROWTH IN THOSE AROUND THEM BECAUSE THESE QUALITIES FLOW FROM WITHIN THEM.

keys! Once you and I put our trust in Christ, it's as if God tells us, "I see you seeing Me! Now I can pour all of Myself into you."

Though my thoughts about myself and my life were once out of proper alignment and disordered—I thought I just needed to get all those plates spinning at once—God's love entered, putting an end to my circus act and giving me peace. No longer do I need to live anxiously, scattering myself all over the place as I try to keep the plates in the air. I know that even if all the plates come crashing down on the floor, He will not be angry with my mess.

We live wholeheartedly when we know that we are totally and completely loved by God and that He wants to bring peace, hope, and beauty to the earth through us, each and every day in every situation. God invites us to join Him as He redeems, restores, and transforms the world by His love. That's wholehearted living—trusting God to strengthen us when we don't feel like we are enough and trusting Him to remove any prideful places in our hearts where we are tempted to build an altar to ourselves.

A life lived wholeheartedly, drawing upon the love of God, leads to true wellness. God calls you to approach your work, your play, your relationships, and even your eating and drinking this way. No matter how messy things might get, His love will lower every hill and raise every valley, so you are free to be fully and wholly you!

Sufficiency

In the 1980s, Frito-Lay launched a marketing campaign for their Lay's potato chips with the taunt "Bet you can't eat just one!" And as a girl who loved a good friendly competition, I heard it as a challenge. When my mom brought the puffy yellow package of chips home from the grocery store, it didn't sit for long. My brother and I grabbed the bag from the pantry, opened it, and told each other, "I bet you can't eat just one!" We went toe-to-toe to see if either of us could eat just one and walk away. And guess what . . . we couldn't. We didn't. I took a crispy, salty, wafer-thin slice of heaven, and as it melted on my tongue,

I passed the bag to my brother. Then he did the same. After that, our adolescent pleasure-seeking brains must have lit up like a pinball machine, and we were all in! We both laughed at being losers, but we didn't care. We just kept fighting over the bag on our way back to the TV room.

Give humans something good, and they have to have more. If a little is good, then a lot must be better, right? Well, not always. On one hand, our insatiable appetite for more and more goodness is God's fingerprint on us, a sign that we are made in His image. After all, He is a good God who makes and gives only what is good. It is no wonder we gravitate toward goodness like a compass is drawn toward true north. On the other hand, this quest for goodness is easily hijacked when we use physical substitutes to satisfy our spiritual cravings. The flesh never knows when to say when. Left to its own reasoning, the flesh always says, "More!"

The definition of *sufficiency* is "the quality or state of being sufficient: adequacy."[11] You experience it when you are comfortably full after eating and have no hunger or want, and when you are able to be satisfied in each moment. In sufficiency, circumstances have no power to define your worth.

When people who are losing weight realize that who they are is who God called them to be, they are set free! When they are sufficiently full after eating, they are satisfied in the moment, and circumstances do not define their feelings of worth. The chains of self-condemnation, doubt, and ridicule no longer have the power to control. The goal of *The Wellness Revelation* is that we would respond to the prompting of God to care for our health, to do the godly thing, to go the better way, and that we would hear the Lord say, "This is sufficient for you." Period. The goal is to recognize that God has made us holy and whole. The goal is *not* a number.

Our God is the God of sufficiency. He is about meeting our needs without giving us everything we want. He knows that if left to our own devices, we would never know when to say, "Enough!" At our core, we are selfish and greedy people. Why do you think Eve believed the lie? So that she and Adam could have what God has. They were not satisfied with *not* having it *all*.

None of us will ever be enough or have enough apart from God. In the words of Bruce Springsteen, "Everybody's got a hungry heart."[12] The vacuum that God has placed in all of our hearts leaves us wanting and seeking more and more. Yet apart from Him, we will never fully be satisfied. Eventually, this leaves us either soft and broken or hard-hearted. The broken and humble in heart can turn to a God who can satisfy. And the hard-hearted are devastated when they fall off the pedestal of self.

The psalmist took this to heart when he wrote, "My flesh and my heart may fail, but God is the strength of my heart and my portion forever" (Psalm 73:26). If you struggle with overeating, you might want to sear this verse into your memory! God's strength is enough for you, and He is your sufficiency.

God wants you holy and whole, which requires you to be mindful and wholehearted as you find your sufficiency in Christ.

THE BATTLE TO BE TRUE

Six months ago I broke my foot. A simple misstep tore one little tendon, which led to significant problems. First, I couldn't walk. Second, a tear in this particular tendon, even a microscopic one like mine, can cause instability in the bones of the big toe and the second toe. Without proper healing, this tear can lead to permanent foot pain and arthritis. My doctor recommended immediate surgery. In a matter of five days, I went from a healthy and strong woman on two feet to one flat on her back as she was wheeled into surgery so doctors could place two rods and a pin in her foot.

In the weeks and months that followed, the medical bills came flooding in. My husband and I couldn't believe that one tiny tendon tear could cost us thousands and thousands of dollars. Just when we thought the bills were all paid off, another one would arrive.

Accidents like my foot injury will happen. But many of the health issues we face today can be avoided if we are proactive—eating whole foods, living wholeheartedly and free of stress because we know we are wholly loved by a holy God—rather than seeking after things we think will give us comfort and pleasure.

It's no secret that the health care system in the United States is under much stress. We are a sick nation living in a wealthy period. We get lots of what we want (rights and resources to pursue happiness) but less of what we need (hearts that are healed and made whole by love, that are set free to set others free). As the cost of health care continues to increase, many of us seem to just go with the flow, praying we won't ever be in medical need even though we may be unable to walk a flight of stairs without becoming winded. Too many of us are versed in reading and speaking the Word, but not in actually living the Word.

Perhaps we've bought into the world's lie about weight loss—that it must be done in the flesh. Voices all around us try to convince us that we simply need to pull ourselves up by our bootstraps and get to work. As believers in Christ, our Rescuer and Redeemer, let's recognize that weight loss is not just a battle of the flesh; it is also a spiritual battle. Just as it would be impossible for you or me to take an orange and separate the fiber from the vitamin C, so we cannot remove pounds from our bodies without first engaging our souls and spirits. The flesh will never be strong enough to fight a war that is greater than itself.

Every Sunday, we sit in the company of the true source of power—God the Almighty—sing His praises, read His words, and nod our heads in agreement. Then we walk out the door and stop looking in the mirror (see James 1:23-24). By claiming our weight as the "cross" we must carry, we miss out on the freedom God has called us to.

Ephesians 6:10-12 tells us where to look for the power we need to live in wholeness and holiness: "Be strong in the Lord and in his mighty power. Put on the full armor of God, so that you can take your stand against the devil's schemes. For our struggle is not against flesh and blood, but against the rulers, against the authorities, against the powers of this dark world and against the spiritual forces of evil in the heavenly realms."

I sense that today the body of Christ is being invited to partner with God on earth in an act of social justice—peace on earth through the bodies of the body of Christ.

Therefore, when Christ came into the world, he said:

"Sacrifice and offering you did not desire,
    but a body you prepared for me;
with burnt offerings and sin offerings
    you were not pleased.
Then I said, 'Here I am—it is written about me in the scroll—
    I have come to do your will, my God.'"

HEBREWS 10:5-7

More than ever, our earth needs healthy and whole people: people who are willing to do God's will in spirit, soul, and body. If we, as followers of Christ, are not being lit on fire to do all we can to agree with God's best for us and to manifest goodness and health in our lives, aren't we just contributing to the problem?

Jesus promised, "You will always have the poor among you" (Mark 14:7, NLT). His Word makes clear that we are to care for them, and our responsibility applies to all forms of poverty—physical, emotional, and spiritual. As far as it depends on us, we are invited to be part of the solution, not the problem.

Now is the time to stand against the adversary's scheme to impoverish our bodies. We can and will prevail, not by our strength, but by God's. Now is the time to let the Scriptures search us, know us, and change us. It's time we burn great amounts of spiritual calories because in Scripture whenever something is sacrificed or sanctified, fire is always involved. Before we make it our business to point out the specks in other people's eyes, we need to deal with the planks in our own.

RESPOND

With All Your Heart

> You're ready! This week as you follow the Wellness Revelation Workout Calendar, you will pick up the pace. Through the videos, you will start moving and applying some of the fitness concepts below, such as cardiovascular and muscular training. Turn to page 240 to access the Wellness Revelation Workout Calendar.

GETTING PHYSICAL

The time has come for us to put some feet to our faith! Let's get moving. The energy required to exercise may seem daunting, especially if you feel you don't have any energy to spare. Please trust me—and even more, trust God—that He will give you just enough to get moving and stay moving. I can guarantee that the amount of energy you spend exercising will come back to you two-fold. Does this seem paradoxical? Much like the Kingdom of God, wouldn't you say?

From this point on, I would like you to rewrite your mental script of why you exercise. I encourage you to perform regular exercise as a time of worship, which, by scriptural definition, involves dedication and sacrifice (see Romans 12:1). Bring your whole self—body, soul, mind, heart, strength, breath, and sweat—dying to your old self and being renewed by God's power and for His glory. Change the focus of your workouts so they center on Him.

In addition to using the Wellness Revelation Workout Calendar, here is a great tip to help turn your workouts from work into worship: Load up your smart phone with your favorite music, including worship songs, and get moving. If you have never considered worship songs as a good motivator, don't knock it till you try it. Or if you are looking for the whole package while you move your feet, consider downloading our free *REVING the Word* podcast workouts. You can find them by searching "Revelation Wellness" on any podcast app or in iTunes. These podcasts will speak God's Word over you as you move your feet to inspirational, upbeat music.

If music isn't your thing and you prefer a quieter and more contemplative route, consider downloading the YouVersion Bible app and reading the verse of the day. Push play on the audio portion of that Scripture, and then during your workout, "chew" on that passage—roll it over in your mind and let it hit your heart as you move your feet. Ask God for revelation as you breathe and move.

You may find that as your physical self is occupied with exercise, you are opening up a new space in your mind where you and the Lord can dwell. This is a *great* time to live out Romans 12:1:

> So here's what I want you to do, God helping you: Take your everyday, ordinary life—your sleeping, eating, going-to-work, and walking-around life—and place it before God as an offering. Embracing what God does for you is the best thing you can do for him.
> THE MESSAGE

Physical exercise is the cornerstone of good and lasting health. Study after study has proven that healthy eating habits and regular exercise are the keys to living longer and with more vitality. They are the *only* true fountain of youth. Sure, you could lose weight simply by eating less. Unfortunately, that approach would only take you so far. It would also be unfair to the rest of you. The inner you would not match the appearance of the healthier outer you. You would still be living as a broken, disconnected, and less-than-whole person.

Your heart will get stronger and stay healthier only with regular cardiovascular exercise. Your muscles will only get and stay stronger through regular resistance training. Remember our battle cry: to love the Lord our God with all our hearts, minds, souls, and strength, and to love others as we love ourselves. We are only as strong as the weakest part of ourselves.

A Stronger Heart

You may notice that you have increased energy from utilizing more whole foods for fuel. Now is a good time to start burning off some stagnant, dormant energy and working your cardiovascular system. Anything that gets your heart rate up for a sustained amount of time qualifies as substantial heart conditioning.

Type: Choose any activity you think you might enjoy. Anything goes! Get physically adventuresome and try different ways to move your body. Dance in your living room. Go outside and walk, run, bike, or hike. Kickbox, punch, swim, or cross-train. (Cross-training engages large muscle groups and all sorts of body movements to increase the heart rate.)

A key thing to consider is your ease of access to the activity you choose. Is it something you can do at home or work? Do you need to go somewhere to participate in the activity, and if so, are you willing to sacrifice that time for the payoff of living well? You certainly can overcome the time barrier, so do not worry. Just be aware. And allow me to encourage you to have some backup activities. Remember, in the end, it's not about the exercise. Moving your body is your spiritual discipline—a space for the *whole* you to connect with the One who insists on moving you toward wholeness and transforming you into more Christlikeness.

It's important that you find an activity you like—a way of moving your body that will energize you, a uniquely designed and impassioned person made in God's image. If you haven't found such an activity yet, pray. Ask God to move you! He most certainly will. While you are waiting for an answer, get rebelliously joyful and wildly obedient and start moving as an act of faith. Movement is your birthright. Take it back!

Frequency: Start with the goal of moving your body at least three times this week. If you are just getting moving, don't overdo it! I often see people whose spirits are willing but whose bodies are not quite up to their "get up and go" zeal. Be kind to yourself as you set and work toward the goal of getting your heart rate up at least three times this week.

If you are already physically active and feel ready for more, go ahead and add a day at a time, a week at a time, working yourself up to six days a week. Always take a day of rest during the week. Your body needs it, and God really likes it. If resting makes you anxious, I bet God would love to talk to you about that—and not while you are moving your body. Sometimes resting is one of the most difficult things we can do. Do it anyway! Stay free.

Time: Ask the Lord to give you the grace to move your body for thirty minutes. This includes warm-up and cooldown time. Does a half hour seem long? It might if you are just rising from the couch. Maybe this will help: Feel free to break up your movement time into two or three mini-sessions throughout your day.

Intensity: This is key! Make your exercise matter. If it's been a while since you deliberately moved your body, establish a steady baseline level of cardiovascular exercise. Go for a thirty-minute walk at a steady pace—heart-pumping but not too strenuous. God will give you the grace, I promise! Just ask Him to walk with you. He's been waiting to do so.

After two weeks or so of establishing a baseline fitness level, you will be ready to start turning up the intensity. On one of your workout days, you might begin incorporating intervals into your thirty minutes of movement. Intervals are set periods of time when you increase your level of exertion beyond what is comfortable before returning to a more relaxed pace. A work interval can last as little as ten seconds and as long as three minutes, with a recovery time equal to or greater than the length of the interval work. An example of a cardiovascular interval session is:

Five-minute warm-up (at a comfortable working pace)

Interval sequence:

> Thirty-second work interval (at an uncomfortable pace) followed by a thirty-second recovery interval (at an easy pace)
> Repeat three times
> Follow with a two-minute steady working pace

Repeat the interval sequence four times

Five-minute cooldown (at a comfortable working pace)

With any increased work effort, be sure to let the Spirit lead you. Have fun as you willingly go into the deeper and harder places the Holy Spirit often uses to release us from the things that hinder us and hold us back.

Continue looking at your workouts as times of worship and freewill offerings to your God. Workouts always cost something, primarily time and energy. How about giving up a little more comfort as well? When your movement time seems to be getting too relaxed, ask the Holy Spirit if it is time to start shaking things up a bit.

Stronger Muscles

When trying to lose weight in a healthy way, resistance training is very important! As you lose weight, you are bound to lose muscle, which is not good. You want to maintain as much muscle on your skeletal frame as possible, since muscle is what keeps your metabolism strong and your body from becoming injured and frail.

Muscle is crucial to a healthy metabolism, the rate at which your body burns calories. The more lean muscle you maintain, the better your metabolism functions even when you are sitting, sleeping, and eating. Think of your body as a furnace. The more muscle you have, the hotter your flame burns. Your metabolism is, to an extent, genetically predetermined. Yet we all have the ability to increase our metabolism by exercise and by resistance training in particular.

When people try to lose weight by eating less and moving more but refuse to resistance train, they end up exchanging quality (lean muscle) for quantity (pounds lost). Let's go for quality!

Your body is most productive and efficient at work when you have a higher muscle-to-fat ratio. Please hear this: *Fat* is not a bad word! God created the body to have and store fat, which helps many of our bodies' processes to continue functioning. Without it, we would die. The amount we carry will vary from person to person.

In addition to boosting your metabolism, resistance training helps preserve bone density since it puts stress on our skeletal frame. We lose bone density every day because of gravity. Yet these minuscule bone losses can be replenished through weight training. It's another paradoxical way in which we have to put ourselves under stress to grow stronger! Resistance training is especially important to anyone who has a family history of osteoporosis, a decrease in bone mass. The accident that most commonly robs elderly people of their independence is a fall that breaks a bone. Resistance training today helps ensure that we will have the muscular strength in the future to keep from falling and have enough bone density to keep a bone from breaking.

Type: You will want to do a total body routine, which is available through many group exercise classes at your local health club.

You might try a circuit style of resistance training as well. This is where small bouts of cardiovascular activity are placed in between resistance exercises so that your heart rate stays up while performing the required strength moves. It is important that each major muscle group (legs, arms, chest, back, abdominals) is trained in each session.

If you'd prefer to complete your resistance training at home, I invite you to go to RevelationWellness.org and check out RevWell TV, our online workout program. It offers hundreds of cardiovascular and resistance training classes designed to strengthen your body while igniting your heart in worship. (Warning: Learning how to turn workouts into acts of worship may wreck your ability to attend a regular fitness class without sensing God's good pleasure, which goes beyond a significant calorie burn. We call this being marvelously ruined.)

Frequency: The American College of Sports Medicine recommends that resistance training be performed at least two times a week and should include all major muscle groups.[13] This means that you need to put your muscles and bones under stress, or overload, by using added weights at least twice a week.

Time: While resistance training is necessary, especially when working to lose weight but not muscle mass, it should take no longer than twenty to forty minutes. Unless you are planning on competing for the next Mr. or Ms. Olympia title, you should not have to spend all day throwing weights around.

Intensity: Resistance training is like cardiovascular exercise in that it should be *challenging*! To avoid wasting time in the gym, make each repetition count and move intentionally. Use good form and the appropriate weight, and keep momentum (the swinging of body parts due to speed) to a minimum.

You will know you are using an appropriate amount of weight if you can perform two sets of ten to twenty repetitions. The last three reps of your second set should begin to challenge you. If time permits, you can add a third set of ten to twenty repetitions. If you can complete all three sets with little to no discomfort, it's time to consider adding weight or incorporating new exercises to challenge your muscles in new ways.

JESUS IS MY PERSONAL TRAINER

When I was a personal trainer, people came to me when they were seeking physical transformation. It's probably fair to say that most of them didn't feel equipped to make the change on their own. They looked to me to tell them what to stop doing and what to start doing to get them to their desired goal.

They also wanted me to hold them accountable. Although my clients told me they wanted to lose weight, gain muscle mass, or look better in a bathing suit, as I've already said, I believe most were seeking the peace of mind they thought would come with getting what they wanted.

We are all looking for peace. We are all wandering east of Eden, and every human heart is trying to get back to the garden space where we walked and talked with God in the cool of the day. And Jesus has blazed the trail, the way for us to get back to the place where all things are as they should be—the place where all is right with ourselves and the world. Only the assurance that we are loved and right with God can give us the peace we are looking for, the peace of mind that six-pack abs can never give.

Knowing we are loved by God enables us to live wholeheartedly and with integrity, just as we are, without waiting for some better version of ourselves to show up. God keeps us whole and upright as we stay underneath the banner of His love.

The two major enemies of loving God, yourself, and others well are pride and unbelief. (Remember the two weight-loss scenarios I shared with you earlier in this chapter?) Whether or not we get what we want, we can easily fall into one or both of these ditches along the road of our freedom to worship God:

Pride: elevating love for ourselves above love for God and others
Unbelief: giving up on loving ourselves, God, and others

Take a moment to assess how your whole heart is doing. Refer to the diagram on the next page, which represents the relationship between you and God. God is love, and you were created to receive His love to meet your daily needs and immeasurably more. But the enemy will do his best to pull you into the ditch of either focusing too much on your own needs and rights (pride) or giving up hope and growing numb (unbelief).

Next get quiet and ask the Father, "How does my pride get in the way of receiving Your love with my whole heart?" Write down every word or action that lines up with pride under the "pride" column. Then ask Him, "How does my unbelief get in the way of accepting and giving Your love with my whole heart?" Again, write down every word or thought that the Holy Spirit brings to mind. Pride and unbelief will prevent you from living a full and free life.

When it comes to training your physical body, a personal trainer can help. But when it comes to teaching your inner person, your spiritual being, Jesus is the best personal trainer. He is most able and willing to correct your form when it comes to loving God, yourself, and others. He can show you what continues to sabotage your ability to live a healthy, whole, free, and upright life.

GOD'S LOVE

Enables Us to Live a Wholehearted,
Righteous, and Justified Life.

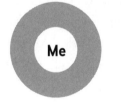

Unbelief   Me   **Pride**

RENEW

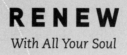

With All Your Soul

Set aside some disciplined and focused time this week to read, study, pray, and apply God's Word to your life.

Strength

1. Read 2 Timothy 1:5-8. What does God's Spirit *not* make us? Describe a time in your life when a timid spirit affected your health and well-being.

2. According to 2 Timothy 1:7, what did God's Spirit give us? How do these God-given attributes change the way you care for your health? How could you apply God's *power* as you work through the Wellness Revelation program? How could you apply God's *love* in this time?

3. This passage also says God gives us self-discipline. Paul uses the Greek word that also means "calling to soundness of mind" and comes from a word meaning "to restore to one's senses." Though our culture tends to view self-discipline as "getting tough," Paul seems to be calling us to clear and restore our minds. Every day we fight for sober, clear thinking in Christ. In what areas of life do you most long for soundness of mind?

Sufficiency

4. Read 2 Corinthians 12:7-9 and then fill in the blank: "My grace is _____ for you." What does sufficiency mean for you? In what way is your battle for health and wholeness *not* just about your weaknesses but about God's strength?

5. Read Exodus 16:13-15. What gift did God give the Israelites in the desert? Read verses 16-18. How much did each person have? Read Exodus 16:4. How did God say He was going to see if they would follow His directions? Finally, read Exodus 16:19-20. What happened to people who took too much? What does this passage tell us about how God provides for us? Why must we trust His provision and timing?

Wholehearted Living

6. Read Romans 6:15-18. Living under the law means claiming righteousness by doing what we are supposed to do and not doing what we are not supposed to do. (Can you sense the mounting pressure of keeping all the plates spinning?) By trying to follow the rules of the law, we hope to earn our right to be seen as acceptable before God and others. Why doesn't this approach work? What happens when we attempt it?

7. Every one of us has "[fallen] short of the glory of God" (Romans 3:23). But grace repeatedly and inexhaustibly puts us back in right relationship with

God because Jesus paid for our whole and free lives. How has grace led you toward a more whole and complete self? Away from a life of fear, shame, and guilt?

8. According Romans 6:16, what leads to our righteousness—wholehearted living—under grace? Why does it have this effect?

9. Without becoming legalistic, and with the knowledge that there is nothing you can do or add to what God has done and who He is, how can you offer your body as a slave to righteousness?

10. According to Galatians 3:11, what must the righteous (the wholehearted) live by?

Dear Jesus,

I know that You came to earth to restore my health and well-being and to make it possible for me to be firmly rooted in You. Thank You that You have never wavered in Your desire to rescue my drowning heart, to heal my broken heart, and to restore and set me free with a whole heart. I believe that You are able to do all that You have promised. Thank You for Your gift of grace, which is stronger than anyone else's strength. Thank You for never giving up on me, Your rebellious child, and for being my strength. To honor You, I lay myself at Your feet, knowing that through the power of grace I will get back on my feet whenever anything knocks me down.
✝ Amen.

RELATE

With All Your Mind and Strength

The following questions are designed to help you apply all you've learned this week to your fitness journey. Get with your accountability partner or small group and work honestly through these questions. Consider journaling your answers with God before sharing with your partner or group.

1. How are you doing with food logging and meal planning? What is the hardest part of maintaining these disciplines? What benefits are you reaping?

2. Have you begun regular exercise at this point? If not, why not? If you have, how is that going?

3. How does the invitation to live a wholehearted life change your vision for achieving a balanced life? What do you think God wishes to remove from your life to help you achieve wholehearted living? What does God want to give you to help you build a wholehearted life? Be as specific as possible.

4. What does the statement "Jesus is my personal trainer" mean to you? Use your imagination. What image does that statement evoke?

RECIPROCATE

Love Greater Than Fear

by Tammy LaFleur,
Revelation Wellness Instructor

Revelation Wellness serves at HopeFest, a citywide outreach in Phoenix that offers free medical, dental, and other services to between fifteen thousand and twenty thousand people in need. Our ministry is there to encourage, entertain, and promote hope and fun through movement and activities. Essentially, Revelation Wellness brings a party to the people who are waiting in line for services. Some people camp out the night before the event to make sure they don't lose their places in line.

I met Sarah the first week we served at HopeFest. Revelation Wellness had set up many activities, including a circuit workout with several stations. We presented a T-shirt and water bottle to participants who completed the circuit. Sarah approached the first station, where I was waiting to lead her through the workout. She seemed tired and sad, yet when she smiled, she beamed.

As we began to go through the stations, I could see that she was becoming more open and that her heart was feeling lighter. Sarah and I approached the boxing station. For this exercise, we use a strike shield that runs the length of my arm for a punching pad. I told Sarah to punch the pad with her right fist. She looked me in the eye and said two words: "I can't." A little stunned, I immediately followed with a confident "Oh yes you can!" This was a natural reaction from me because I believe strongly that with God nothing is impossible.

The next thing Sarah said literally knocked the wind out of me. "No, I can't. I don't punch. I get punched."

She gets punched? My heart began pounding. I wanted to stop, hold her, and tell her everything was going to be okay. Instead, I looked her straight in the eyes and said, "Well, today you will fight back." By God's mercy and His great love, she believed it. Sarah began with a timid and gentle punch, but as I encouraged her to fight harder, her punches became stronger and stronger. As she punched, I told her how deeply she was loved and cared for by the Lord, that He desired to protect her, that He had not left her, and that He was waiting for her.

Sarah began to cry as she punched, and it was clear that something in her spirit had shifted. I hugged her tightly and prayed over her words of life and the promises of the Father. There was no need to finish the stations. The purpose of Sarah stepping into that circuit workout had been accomplished. She had encountered the love of God, and she was transformed in that moment. As I handed Sarah her "LOVE > fear" T-shirt and water bottle, she cried some more. Then we prayed before hugging and saying good-bye.

The following year, the Revelation Wellness team returned to bring love to the people at HopeFest once again. I was overjoyed when I saw Sarah coming toward me, smiling and beaming. She had her children with her, and she exuded the joy of a proud mama.

Sarah told me how her life had turned around completely since HopeFest the year before. Every morning she would wake up and see that water bottle on her kitchen sink. She began to vow to make daily decisions for herself and her children based on love and not on fear. Sarah took steps to file a restraining order against her ex-husband. She expressed how hard this was because she had feared him for so long. Sarah obtained full custody of her children, got a new job, and moved into a new home with her kids. She said that she now knows the love of God and that His love is greater than any fear. This truth gave her the courage to take the necessary steps toward change.

I am incredibly humbled to have been a part of Sarah's story. God uses the ministry of Revelation Wellness to change lives. We offer the hope only found in Jesus to those who are without hope. It is not primarily about the fitness, but about His love healing the broken. I will never forget that day and cannot wait to see what the Lord will do at the next HopeFest. His love never quits!

RENEW YOUR MIND

We demolish arguments and every pretension that sets itself up against the knowledge of God, and we take captive every thought to make it obedient to Christ.

2 CORINTHIANS 10:5

For the last two weeks, we have focused on two critical goals when improving our health—eating less and moving more. We can't deny their importance when seeking wellness and wholeness. This week, however, we are going to go deeper and discover how we can make a positive shift in our hearts and minds, which will affect our relationships with God, ourselves, other people, and even our circumstances. Renewing our thoughts and attitudes is critical if we are to stand strong when our initial enthusiasm over changing our eating and exercise habits begins to wane. Even more important, we will never achieve the wellness and wholeness God wants for us until we rest in our identity as His children—and that starts in our hearts and minds.

As a mother of two, I am in love with my children. From the day Jack and Sophia were born, I knew I would do anything to ensure the safety and satisfaction of their hearts. When they are healthy, whole, and free to chase their dreams, I am one happy mama bear. Still, if I am not careful, as a flawed and fearful mama in the flesh, I can do too much to make my children happy. My love for my children is flawed because I am flawed. But God, our good, good Father, has perfect love for His kids. He gives only good gifts to us. As Jesus said, "Which of you fathers, if your son asks for a fish, will give him a snake instead? Or if he asks for an egg, will give him a scorpion? If you then, though you are evil, know how to give good gifts to your children, how much more will your Father in heaven give the Holy Spirit to those who ask him!" (Luke 11:11-13).

The heart of God, our Father, is partial toward His children. He bends His ears to hear us. When you ask Him to help you get healthy, whole, and free, His answer is a big fat *yes*! What father wouldn't want a sound mind and a spirit of power and love for his kids, that they might know who they are and how they are designed to add good to the world? Not a good father. But we have a good, good Father who says, "Yes and amen!" to these requests. "No matter how many promises God has made, they are 'Yes' in Christ" (2 Corinthians 1:20).

You might think that your heart is the engine of your body. In purely physical terms, that is true. The heart is the muscle that pumps the blood needed to keep your body in business. Mechanically speaking, the heart is your motor. Without your heartbeat, you would cease to exist.

However, when it comes to moving your desires and intentions forward, your mind takes on that function. The desires of your heart are like fuel that must be fed into an engine (your mind), or your life will constantly backfire. You might have the best intentions. For example, you might long for a close relationship with your family, wish for a more fulfilling vocation, or desire more energy and vitality. But unless your mind becomes convinced to act on these intentions, your goals will be as useless as gasoline poured into a car with a burned-out motor.

The same is true in our relationship with God: He can be working in our hearts, but if our minds aren't being changed as well, we may not make as much progress as we'd like. I don't know about you, but when my heart finally awakened to the good news that God not only loves me but really likes me, I spent a few years feeling as if I were losing my mind. God's Word was transforming my heart, but I still faced the same old circumstances—an unraveling marriage, extended family members who were battling addictions, and friends and family who didn't know what to do with me now that I was freaking out on Jesus. My heart was new, but my mind . . . my mind was frozen stuck. In my heart, I received the Word with great joy, but my day-to-day feelings about my circumstances were infected by my diseased mind. Unbeknownst to me, I needed a mind transplant to go along with my heart transplant.

This became particularly clear to me one day when my husband, Simon, and I were not getting along. Though I don't remember all the details, it was

Remember to use your Moving Forward Journal this week to track your food and water intake, as well as to remain focused on this week's Scripture verse. You can download a copy at www.revelationwellness.org/book/workout or photocopy the template on page 239.

most likely because I felt as if he did not love me the way I deserved or the way Jesus loved me. My feelings were hurt, and my husband was passive—our usual standoff pattern. Earlier in the day we had promised our kids that we would take them to dinner, so we headed off to one of their favorite restaurants. The usual stench of bitter, stale air filled the car between Simon and me. The kids seemed to have no clue that their mama's heart was on lockdown because she was convinced she was being abandoned, while their daddy's heart was growing weary from the shame of sensing that he was never able to get it right.

I remember walking into that restaurant feeling as if I were wearing a thousand-pound suit of armor. But even as tired as I was, there was no way I was going to take off my protective gear and risk further hurt.

As the hostess seated us, I humphed and slid down heavily into our booth. While the kids colored, Simon and I sat without speaking. Slowly the kids began to pick up on our lack of energy, and they, too, got quiet. The silence was deafening, and it made me sick to my stomach. *God, this is not what You promised me! Where are You?* I yelled in my mind.

Just then a woman holding the hand of a little girl approached our table. She wore a big, kind smile and walked like a queen. "Hello, I'm Maggie," she said sweetly, "and this is Emma." Emma was one of my son's favorite friends from school. Every day after school, Jack had been telling me lovely little stories about Emma. Up until this point, I had only seen her from afar on the playground. This was a much-needed surprise in a very tense moment.

Overcome with joy, I stood up quickly, extended my hand as if I had been struck by lightning, and jovially said, "Oh my goodness! It's so great to meet you!"

Maggie and I had a warm exchange about our kids, their school, their interests, and their blossoming friendship. My face went from a frown to a smile so fast that it got a cramp. What sticks with me most is how quickly I was transported from a world of dread, hopelessness, hurt, and despair into a world of fun, wonder, joy, delight, and laughter. While talking with Maggie, I felt as if I were floating on air.

Finally Maggie and Emma, still hand in hand, walked away. Something happened next that I will never forget. I slid back into that brown pleather booth as if I had just been handed a prison sentence. I went from walking on air to feeling the weight of despair in less than a second flat. Right then I had an "aha" moment. As if I were the coyote in *The Road Runner Show*, an anvil of revelation fell on my head.

What's wrong with me? I screamed inside. *That woman who was just talking with Maggie . . . that is who I really am. That's the true me! I am that woman! I want to be that woman! God, help me!*

From inside of me, God's voice rose up and said, *Yes. That is who you are. And we are getting there.* I realized God was asking me to surrender my mind so He could give it back to me—new and more powerful than ever before.

Our minds have the potential to harness a tremendous amount of transforming power. In Romans 12:2, the apostle Paul reminds us how we are to filter our minds' strength: "Do not conform to the pattern of this world, but be transformed by the *renewing* of your mind. Then you will be able to test and approve what God's will is——his good, pleasing and perfect will" (emphasis mine).

Transform is defined as making "a thorough or dramatic change in the form, appearance, or character of."[14] *To be transformed.* Who doesn't want that? If you have joined this program, I bet that you are looking for some type of change. Maybe you are hoping to take dramatic before-and-after pictures like the ones you've seen online or in magazines (even though you are convinced they've been Photoshopped!).

The truth of the matter is that as much as God should be our sufficiency, we still tend to seek affirmation for who we are and how we appear in the eyes of others. I strongly urge you *not* to seek transformation for the approval of others. This is a quick way to a dead end! You must desire change for God and from God alone, for His glory and for your joy.

The kind of transformation Jesus offers us is not found in endless time on a treadmill or months of strict eating. Those are old patterns of our dead way of life, conformed to the world. Through faith, we now have access to a powerful, transformative way of life that reveals God's glory. We can continually breathe the air of heaven through His Word. He gives us the permission and power to remain free even when the enemy attacks our minds and tries to steal our joy and our identity as His royal children. We all are offered the power to transform ourselves and our circumstances—but first it will cost us our minds.

THE BATTLEGROUND

Tucked into the middle of Paul's letter to the Romans is a passage that reads much like the 1938 Abbott and Costello routine "Who's on First?" It explains why you probably feel as if you are losing your mind as you gain your new life in Christ. Read it slowly, carefully, and repeatedly if you have to.

> I do not understand what I do. For what I want to do I do not do, but what I hate I do. And if I do what I do not want to do, I agree that the law is good. As it is, it is no longer I myself who do it, but it is sin living in me. For I know that good itself does not dwell in me, that is, in my sinful nature. For I have the desire to do what is good, but I cannot carry it out. For I do not do the good I want to do, but the evil I do not want to do—this I keep doing. Now if I do what I do not want to do, it is no longer I who do it, but it is sin living in me that does it.
>
> So I find this law at work: Although I want to do good, evil is right there with me. For in my inner being I delight in God's law; but I see another law at work in me, waging war against the law of my mind and making me a prisoner of the law of sin at work within me. What a wretched man I am! Who will rescue me from this body that is subject to death? Thanks be to God, who delivers me through Jesus Christ our Lord!
>
> So then, I myself in my mind am a slave to God's law, but in my sinful nature a slave to the law of sin.
>
> ROMANS 7:15-25

And there you have it! Paul was honestly exposing himself, his short-comings, and the struggles that he faced, just like the rest of us. We all fall into patterns of doing what we ought *not* to do, even when we know what we ought *to* do.

From a worldly perspective, you can see how we might fall victim to the vicious cycle of (1) wanting to do good, (2) picking ourselves up and making efforts to change, (3) falling short of our good intentions or even slipping up, (4) beating ourselves up, and (5) retreating back to the place of comfort by giving up. Round and round we go! How utterly defeating.

But "thanks be to God . . . through Jesus Christ our Lord!" In facing the reality that we all fall short of the glory of God, we are called to put on our spiritual armor and enter back into the battle, for God is *with* us and *for* us.

The battle for our health—like so much in our lives—will take place in our minds.

Though we live in the world, we do not wage war as the world does. The weapons we fight with are not the weapons of the world. On the contrary, they have divine power to demolish strongholds. We demolish arguments and every pretension that sets itself up against the knowledge of God, and we take captive every thought to make it obedient to Christ. And we will be ready to punish every act of disobedience, once your obedience is complete.

2 CORINTHIANS 10:3-6

The mind is the battleground between God and the sin that separates us from Him, ourselves, and others. As long as we are willing to renew our minds according to His Word, God will be the ultimate victor there. Because we are God's children and created in His image, we are easily inspired to do the right things. Our hearts then supply the fuel, or the motive, to follow Christ.

Then, however, each good intention must make it past the battleground of our minds. Too often, we quickly wave the white flag of surrender there. When we see the seemingly insurmountable obstacles foisted upon us by our enemy—the flaming arrows of doubt, disbelief, discouragement—we turn tail and run.

In such moments, we have surrendered to the wrong party! We must construct walls around the battlegrounds of our minds to protect us from the flaming arrows of doubt. If we don't, we will be full of "would have, should have, could have" regrets. We must remember, too, that God's Word often fills our hearts with passionate fuel that burns for Him and makes us willing to follow Him into the deep places where we are in way over our heads. Unless God took us into impossible situations and circumstances where He must prove the truth of His Word, when would we give Him credit or the world give Him glory?

Because our minds are battlefields, we must study the mind of Christ and pattern our thoughts after His. After all, we are created in His image. First Corinthians 2:16 says, "'Who has known the mind of the Lord so as to instruct him?' But we have the mind of Christ."

As the apostle Paul makes clear in his letter to the Corinthians, we will never fully understand God. However, Scripture reveals some characteristics of the mind of Christ, including three attributes we need to develop as we continue on our wellness journey.

Understanding and Wisdom

God has complete understanding of who we are and what His purposes are for our lives.

> The Lord is the everlasting God,
>   the Creator of the ends of the earth.
> He will not grow tired or weary,
>   and his understanding no one can fathom.

ISAIAH 40:28

Our minds do best when we fill them with wisdom by seeking to understand who God is. That's contrary to the world's view of wisdom as something we can gain through study and education. In America, we start out with our ABCs and might go all the way to a PhD. With study and time, we gain more and more knowledge. If we get a PhD in a particular field, we are considered wise in that field. This is a linear, systematic approach toward wisdom. However, as with almost everything, if you want to understand God, you need to flip the world's system upside down.

Psalm 111:10 says, "The fear of the LORD is the beginning of wisdom; all who follow his precepts have good understanding." God does not care much about what school you went to, or how many of the Bible's sixty-six books you have memorized. To get a true understanding of God, you must first fear Him.

We don't like the word *fear*. It's another four-letter word, and it conjures up an image of someone trembling in the corner while facing imminent danger. Relating this type of fear to a loving God doesn't seem to make sense, and it doesn't. That is not what God is looking for from His people. That kind of fear comes from an orphan spirit, like a child who has grown up on the streets, fending for him- or herself and unable to rely on a loving parent.

The fear of the Lord is more like the healthy fear I want my own children to have around fire. In my Phoenix neighborhood, fall is the time to lock up our backyard pools and pull out our fire pits. I love sitting in front of our house in an Adirondack chair, stoking the orange glow inside an iron bowl as the heat covers my body like a blanket. There's something about the dancing flames, the sounds of crackling and popping, and the warmth that seems to draw all the neighbors, young and old. As much as I want my kids to join me and our friends by the fire pit, I would never allow them to carelessly run around it as they show me their latest ninja skills! I taught my children to fear and respect the fire so they can enjoy it as beautiful and beneficial without getting hurt. So it is with the fear of the Lord. In fact, God describes Himself using that very same image: "The LORD your God is a consuming fire, a jealous God" (Deuteronomy 4:24).

Godly fear stems from our awareness that, through our sin, we have carelessly danced around the fire and gotten burned but that His love can heal us. This godly fear reminds us that no matter how hard we try to do what we ought, we still do the things we ought not to do. This is why God sent His Son.

In my opinion, other religions fall short of the full redemption and freedom story because they stop at respect, and they operate in fear. They do not encourage followers to seek the intimacy that comes from knowing God. Our faith is not a religion. It is a relationship, and Jesus desires intimacy with us. Just as He wants us to share everything on our hearts, we desire to understand not only who God is, but what He does, how He thinks, what He feels, what makes Him happy, and what makes Him sad. Ultimately, what makes Him happy makes us happy too.

The more we grow in understanding of and intimacy with Christ, the more we will know who we are and be freed to grow into our true, whole selves. This is why God's Word tells us, "The beginning of wisdom is this: Get wisdom. Though it cost all you have, get understanding" (Proverbs 4:7).

An Undivided Mind

Not only is God's mind filled with all wisdom and knowledge, it is also undivided. Unlike our minds, which easily change course depending on our thoughts and feelings, God never changes His mind. His love for us will always be the same.

Our minds are easily distracted and deceived—even when we're doing something we love. I have a confession to make. I really like to work! If something needs to get done, I'm your gal! A ringing phone and e-mails in my in-box excite me, reminding me that I am needed and can use my gifts to keep things moving. But here's the problem—after a while, all the alerts, dings, and bells slowly steal my joy and kill my hope. I sometimes feel like prey that has been caught in a trap and is being pecked to death by a deranged chicken! I need more peace and wholeness in a world that seems to be pulling me in countless directions.

So how do we keep our minds undivided and whole? By taking all our thoughts captive to Christ—simple in theory but hard to do. It's something we have to keep practicing. Since we are human, emotions often rise up inside us, threatening to jump past the peace and presence of the Lord within us and head straight into the battleground of our minds. A mind at war is immediately divided within itself. That is why we must pay attention to our thought lives.

How do we do that? Second Corinthians 10:5 tells us that "we demolish arguments and every pretension that sets itself up against the knowledge of God, and we take captive every thought to make it obedient to Christ." That requires intentionality, and the practical application is this: *You must slow down!*

I think that as Christians, we are really good at throwing Bible verses at bad thoughts, but we never get to the root of where those accusations come from. They are like criminals running loose in the streets of our minds. They need a day in court! Take a moment to slow down, put that thought in handcuffs, and make it stand trial. Ask God, "Father, what do *You* think about this thought? Where did this thought come from? What would *You* like me to do about _____, which is causing me to feel _____?" We can't go wrong if we seek God's authority on all matters, especially when we get stuck and find ourselves—rather than the enemy whom Christ defeated—in handcuffs. We will know the truth and the truth will keep us free.

Taking our thoughts captive requires practice, practice, practice. We have to learn to slow down and see the warning signs that our minds are beginning to divide. We can minimize or avoid the carnage in ourselves and others if we take all our thoughts, lay them at His feet, and wait for clarity. Let Christ be your example.

Christ is meek. In this world, we often think *meek* equals *weak*, but that is incorrect. One definition of *meekness* is "strength under control." Christ carried our sins on His blameless back, and not once did He decide His suffering wasn't worth it or rage against the world's injustice toward Him. Amidst the criticism, the naysayers, and the haters, Jesus stayed the course. As a result, the enemy lost the ultimate battle, and we have won! Christ was, and is, the embodiment of a quiet strength. We need this meekness of mind, this strength under control— even when we experience pain.

God knows that without seasons of suffering, we would begin to forget who He is and what He has done. If we experienced only comfort and ease, slowly but surely we would wander from Him and lose our wonder of Him. God uses our suffering to keep us sensitive to His presence and to make us more like Christ. He also demonstrates His love, strength, and power through our unfailing love and devotion toward Him in difficult circumstances. So, friends, count it all joy when you find yourselves in the middle of a battle, and keep taking all your thoughts captive to Christ (see James 1:2, NKJV; 2 Corinthians 10:3-5). When we do so, God wins, we get an undivided mind, and God gets His glory. We can't lose.

Freedom from Fear, Worry, Anxiety, and Uncertainty

God also permits pain in our lives because living under tension can help build us up and make us more like Christ. For a personal trainer, tension is a necessary evil. In fact, the whole point of hiring a personal trainer is to help you identify those weaknesses (either in your habits or in your body) that are keeping you from experiencing progress and achieving your goals. The trainer then helps develop a program designed to target your weaknesses by subjecting them to some form of tension. If your goal is to increase your upper body strength, the tension may come from a new regimen of push-ups. If you want to be able to resist temptation when a coworker brings in a plate of home-baked cookies, you must learn to live with the tension that comes with choosing to abstain.

Like a personal trainer, our Father wants to increase our strength to remain faithful rather than fretful, even when we face temptations that regularly cause us to stumble. God works through all of our challenging circumstances to "train" our weaknesses so He can increase our strength and make us more holy and whole.

Losing a job, for instance, interrupts our peace of mind. Not long after we get a pink slip, our minds begin imagining our families without a home, in a shelter, hungry and poor. If we feel a lump on our bodies or see blood in unexpected places, we must quickly fight the "what-ifs" that keep popping into our minds. God, on the other hand, is not anxious, worried, or sitting in heaven wringing His hands wondering how everything is going to work out. He is at complete peace and lacks nothing.

How quickly we humans can go to a place of fear or worry. We start working, toiling, and making plans for our protection and provision. When we worry, we divide ourselves from the peace, protection, and provision of the Father. *Worry* is related to the Old High German word meaning "to strangle." Satan searches for any opportunity to get close enough to reach out with his scaly, cold hands and strangle us. His goal is to steal our life and darken our light. We must protect ourselves from fear, worry, anxiety, uncertainty, and all similar emotions.

Ultimately, worry leads to separation from God, and that makes us more likely to sin—to think, feel, and act in ways that are not godly. In Matthew 6, Jesus explains why we should avoid it:

Do not worry, saying, "What shall we eat?" or "What shall we drink?" or "What shall we wear?" . . . But seek first his kingdom and his righteousness, and all these things will be given to you as well. Therefore do not worry about tomorrow, for tomorrow will worry about itself. Each day has enough trouble of its own.

(VERSES 31, 33-34)

Do you see that Jesus is telling us not to get ahead of ourselves? Don't live tomorrow today. The solution for worry is a mind that is present in this moment and resting in God's love.

Jesus isn't saying we should let life happen willy-nilly or that we should be thoughtless about our lives. Plans are good; after all, "God is not a God of disorder but of peace" (1 Corinthians 14:33). But when our plans do not come together as we hoped, our worry and frantic planning may strangle the life out of us.

Worry exacts a higher cost than loss of sleep. To date, science has proven that stress negatively affects our health and is related to the leading causes of death.[15] Because God loves us and is always for us, He reminds us that we need not worry or have fear. God offers us a better way: We are to give Him all our cares and worries. His Word says, "Cast all your anxiety on him because he cares for you" (1 Peter 5:7).

RENEWAL

Transformation, Paul told the Romans, requires renewing our minds. When we renew something, we give fresh life to it. We get a do-over. God knows that when left alone, we wear ourselves out and fall back into sinful patterns like foolishness, a divided mind, and worry. Yet when we return to our senses, He renews us and gives us a fresh start every time. So how do we renew our minds?

Seek

One way we can renew our minds is simple but requires great discipline. It is by desiring to look for God wherever we go, wherever we are. Think of a mall directory with its red dot and the words "You are here." Likewise, we need the reminder that wherever we go, there God is too.

Seeking God is hard for us because we often shift into autopilot to get through the tasks of the day. Yet I encourage you to look for God wherever you go. Not only is He in you, He is in all places, everywhere. He is the author of all creation. Wherever you see His creation, you see the hands of God: "The heavens declare the glory of God; the skies proclaim the work of his hands" (Psalm 19:1).

The next time you are having a nothing-special kind of day, I dare you to try the following—throw off the nothing-special lens you are looking through and ask God to give you eyes to see what He sees. It's like playing a game of hide-and-seek with God. God loves to hide in people, places, and circumstances because those who seek Him will find—and they will have fun finding Him and be rewarded when they do (see Hebrews 11:6).

Once as I was driving my kids to school, my then eight-year-old son, Jack, said, "Mom, I think you can look at anything and tell me about God." We all laughed, and then my kids began putting me through my paces. First, they asked what I saw when I looked at a tree. I told them I saw God's promise that He would grow me into a tree for the display of His splendor. My son thought he could stump me when he asked me what I saw when I looked at a car tire. After a moment of searching my heart, I told him it reminded me that God's love keeps going and going. It never gives up, blows up, or wears out. When I saw a woman walking to the bus stop, I said, "That is a woman of great nobility, character, and promise—a woman who is God's best."

Ephesians 6 tells us about the battle we are in and urges us to dress appropriately by putting on the breastplate of righteousness, the helmet of salvation, the belt of truth, and the shoes of peace, with God's Word in one hand and the shield of faith in the other (see verses 6:10-18). If I were to add one more important item of war-fashion accoutrement, it would be a pair of goggles. Not the kind you wear swimming or skiing, but the kind aviators like the Wright brothers and Amelia Earhart wore in the early days of flight.

Goggles were essential for early aviators because they protected their eyesight and gave them a clear view of what was going on around them. So it is for us! To keep fighting the good fight and holding on to our identity as children of God, we need to fix our gaze on Him and keep our gospel goggles strapped on tight. If we take them off before we look in the mirror, we will be tempted to call ourselves ugly. If we forget to put them on when we walk into a dark moment, we will run away in fear instead of seeing the light that shines at our feet. If we don't have them on when we survey the landscape, we will conclude that it is disgusting, defiled, and hopeless.

Instead of opting for a pair of rose-colored lenses—the kind of fashionable glasses a woman lounging by the pool and taking life at a leisurely pace would wear—choose to strap on a pair of gospel goggles. Sure, they aren't as sexy as the rose-colored spectacles, but you aren't a person of leisure; you are a foot soldier of hope! What you seek, you will find.

When your goggles are on, you will seek and find that the woman who cut in front of you in line is God's child too. You will see the hurt in that grumpy next-door neighbor who never smiles and always seems angry, and you will hear the Voice of Love prompting you to speak a kind word to him.

I have discovered a secret remedy for my heart on the days I feel all alone, dry, and in need of God's touch. It is found in strapping on those gospel goggles and seeking someone to whom I can give what I myself need. If I long for God's presence, I seek someone to whom I can wholeheartedly give my presence. If I need God's encouragement, I seek someone whom I can encourage.

We are all connected and all in need. Wherever you go, God is there. The Kingdom is always at hand "so that [people] would seek him and perhaps reach out for him and find him, though he is not far from any one of us" (Acts 17:27). Renew your mind first by looking, for then you will find Him.

Wonder

Every year during the high heat of summer, our family rolls out of Phoenix to escape the big fireball in the sky and heads west toward the sea. Summer vacation doesn't officially begin until we have seen that same fireball turn into a glowing orb of orange and set into the Pacific Ocean. As I gaze out into the vastness of a sky so blue it looks as if it were painted by Paul Cézanne, my resting heart rate drops by ten beats or so. In that moment, surrounded by breathtaking beauty and fresh salty air, my childlike wonder is restored.

Interestingly enough, when my husband and I were first married, we lived by that same sea, but I can count on one hand the times we intentionally set off to be inspired by the wonder of the oceanic beauty surrounding us. The daily grind stole our willingness to wonder and play.

A heart that doesn't like to wonder in God will likely wander from Him. Our desire for fresh things often comes at the cost of losing our appreciation for the familiar. A piece of artwork that we once looked at with great awe slowly loses its ability to take our breath away. We play a song, which once made us jump up and dance or that seemed to tell our story, over and over until the day we decide we can't listen to it one more time. The new becomes familiar and eventually gets filed away like a stock image in our brains.

Another path to renewing our minds is seeking to see things from a new perspective. Keep asking God what He is trying to reveal to you, even in those difficult circumstances when you feel overwhelmed. You won't feel lost in drudgery and dejection when you respond to God's greatness with astonishment and when you desire more of what He wants for your life. Our minds are renewed when we, like the apostle Paul, pray "that the God of our Lord Jesus Christ, the glorious Father, may give [us] the Spirit of wisdom and revelation, so that [we] may know him better" (Ephesians 1:17).

Practice the art of wonder as often as possible. Avoid being quick to try to figure everything out. Leave space for the unknown, and use your imagination. Our imaginations get a bad rap; when we use them, the world often says we are simply foolish or childish. But Jesus is clear that only those who are like little children will enter the Kingdom.

Anytime we approach God, we should bring our imaginations. Not only does God love to recreate with us—to spend time with us when we go for a hike, play tennis, or dance—He loves to *re*-create with us. He loves to infuse ordinary situations with His presence and *re*-create them into extraordinary, head-scratching, wonderful places to be.

Have you read the book of Revelation lately? It's hard to read some passages without feeling a sense of wonder:

The horses and riders I saw in my vision looked like this: Their breastplates were fiery red, dark blue, and yellow as sulfur. The heads of the horses resembled the heads of lions, and out of their mouths came fire, smoke and sulfur.

REVELATION 9:17

So go ahead . . . continually train your sense of wonder in the presence of the King. He wants to use you to make the extraordinary happen here on earth.

Read His Word

God also renews us with His Word because His words are alive. Day to day, in every moment, His Word has the ability to actively inspire and refresh our thinking. If the thoughts swirling around in our minds are not in line with God's heart for us, His Word in us waits for our permission to take out the trash. This is why it is important that we don't just seek God in His Word for how He makes us feel. Our thoughts and feelings must submit to what He says: "My child, pay attention to my words; listen closely to what I say. Don't ever forget my words; keep them always in mind. They are the key to life for those who find them; they bring health to the whole body. Be careful what you think, because your thoughts run your life" (Proverbs 4:20-23, NCV).

God's Word is a mirror that you can hold up to see yourself as you are at any time. You can open up His message and gain wisdom and understanding. When your thoughts are anchored in what God has said and what He wants for your life, you can walk confidently in the assurance that if God said it, He will do it.

When my feelings are hurt by what my husband does or doesn't do, my emotions are quick to kick the Holy Spirit out of the driver's seat and take over. God's love for me, spoken to me through His Word, enables me to put a quick end to the joyride of the thief who came to kill, steal, and destroy.

"All Scripture is God-breathed and is useful for teaching, rebuking, correcting and training in righteousness" (2 Timothy 3:16). I love that term—*God-breathed*. The same image is used in the first book of the Bible: "The LORD God formed a man from the dust of the ground and breathed into his nostrils the

A HEART THAT DOESN'T LIKE TO WONDER IN GOD
WILL LIKELY WANDER FROM HIM.

breath of life, and the man became a living being" (Genesis 2:7). God created us through the power of His breath. How intimate! God used just two physical acts when creating all that is: He spoke and He breathed. Everything in creation, except man and woman, He spoke into being. But when it came to us—to those He wanted to make in His own likeness—He came so very close to us, giving us a life kiss. And so began the romance that He knew would break His heart. He watched us fall away into the brokenness of living unholy lives, but He would not leave us broken. A Rescuer, our Savior who put on flesh, was coming.

Still today, our hearts fail and we need CPR for our souls. The "mouth to mouth" that brings us back to life is found in Scripture's 66 books, 1,189 chapters, 31,102 verses, and about 775,000 words. It is important that we find the time to be in the Word, to become familiar with the mind of Christ so that we can transform into more Christlikeness as we begin living a supernatural lifestyle.

Pray

Thinking things out works well when it comes to concrete matters. If you wanted to add a room onto your house, you could go to the Internet to learn all about home construction or to find a contractor who already has that knowledge and could think it out for you.

Trying to think through spiritual matters often leads to further confusion since there are no formulas—only a relationship with the One who created us. Prayer is a means of building that relationship. When I'm lonely, I don't need to understand how Christ's love heals my sadness; as I begin shifting my thoughts toward His love for me through prayer, I find that His presence comforts and encourages me. The only intellect involved is my acute awareness that my thoughts are powerful and can easily hold me captive, away from His presence and love. This is why we must be careful what we think because our thoughts run our lives (see Proverbs 4:23). We need more than just thinking; we need prayer—an ongoing, intimate conversation with God.

Prayer is conversation with God, our friend and our Father. We can tell Him anything. In fact, that's what He is hoping for. What daddy doesn't love to hear his children tell him about their day, or better yet, have his child ask him what he thinks? (If you're the parent of a teenager or an adult, you know what I mean!) There's no warmer feeling in my mama heart than when my teenage kids want to converse with me or get my advice. Oh, the pain we want our kids to avoid by being willing to glean from our wisdom. And think how small our knowledge is compared to that of our heavenly Father!

Yes, God loves to talk with His kids.

In prayer, we share the concerns of our hearts and minds with our heavenly Father so He can help. Even as we are waiting for things to change, simply being able to talk with Him about it can help tremendously. When I begin to pray, I am entering into the very presence of God Himself. Even though He already knows my heart and needs, He loves to hear me speak.

In Mark 11:24, Jesus makes an amazing promise: "Whatever you ask for in prayer, believe that you have received it, and it will be yours." What a great reminder that God loves us and wants to give us fullness of life. Anything that troubles us, worries us, or keeps us up at night has no lasting power. God, our good Father, will act on our behalf. And while we wait for Him to act, we get the peace and presence of God Himself—the Everlasting Father, Prince of Peace, Wonderful Counselor, and Mighty God (see Isaiah 9:6).

You might wonder, though, why some things you pray for never seem to happen. Notice what Mark 11:25 says: "When you stand praying, if you hold anything against anyone, forgive them, so that your Father in heaven may forgive you your sins." God cares more about changing the condition of your heart than about changing your circumstances.

A mind filled with contempt, revenge, or bitterness is not aligned with God's. And if our hearts (the fuel) and minds (the engines) are in alignment with His will, we will come to realize that some things we asked for in prayer (that weren't in alignment with His will or timing) have been withheld for our own good. So as you pray, don't hold grudges against others or God. Trust that He knows best and He uses all things for your good.

Pray when you are tempted and pray when you are thankful. Pray for others, to take your focus off yourself, but do ask for what you need and then believe that God will give you His very best. God doesn't mind if you repeat yourself. Get into the habit of praying as much as you can, for as long as you can. Even if your circumstances don't seem to change overnight, you are likely to be amazed at the results. As Oswald Chambers wrote, "To say that 'prayer changes things' is not as close to the truth as saying, 'Prayer changes *me* and then I change things.'"[16]

Being in an ongoing communicative relationship with God is one of our greatest delights as His children. We get to talk with God. We get to listen to Him. And He is always speaking. Sometimes as we read His Word, we are brought naturally into His living presence, where we talk with our small group (the Father, Son, and Holy Spirit) about His message and how it is colliding with our lives. And sometimes we just climb up on our Father's lap, snuggle in, and let His love transform us—no mental gymnastics involved. Prayer is relational proximity to God. How close are you willing to go?

Believe

Do you know that every person we meet in the New Testament who came to Jesus for healing was healed? Every one. God does not show favoritism. He is a lover of faith! In Matthew 9:20, a woman reached out and touched Jesus' cloak because she *believed* He could heal her. And because of her belief, He did. Seven verses later, we read that Jesus healed two blind men who had faith He could heal them.

What kind of amazing God is this? All we need to do is believe in what He can do, and it will be done? Jesus wasn't patronizing us when He commanded us to have faith like a child's. It's as if Jesus is saying, "Your grown-up brains, with their schooling, reasoning, and maturity, are nice and all, but sometimes they get in the way of the Way. Remember when you were a little kid and believed anything that someone you trusted told you? Yeah, you need to respond to Me in that same way."

Take time to ask yourself, *Do I believe? Do I believe that God desires me to be healthy and whole? Do I believe that He is strong enough to help me hold on when I am weak and tempted?* It is okay to wrestle with these questions. Because of our human condition, we are always in a tug-of-war between belief and unbelief. We must not feel shame over our unbelief, but we must take that battle to the Lord.

As you seek to grow in your faith, don't fall into the second trap, which is to have faith only "because God said to." Because He is God, He could have made us love Him because He said to. But what kind of love would that be? Love is love only when it is given and chosen freely. Fear-based faith wouldn't lead to a relationship but to a dictatorship.

Believing only "because God said to" will lead to our salvation but not to our transformation. A faith-filled life with God challenges us to remember the truth that God wanted us, He chose us, He knows us, He hears us, He sees us, and He is committed to loving us with the utmost fidelity. God is who He says He is, He hears us when we cry, and He acts on our behalf in accordance with His will.

God loves faith. Faith moves God, and God moves mountains!

RESPOND

With All Your Heart

Be sure to access the Wellness Revelation Workout Calendar on page 240.
This week you will work on increasing your flexibility,
as well as your ability to be still and know.

I t is now time to exercise your mind as you exercise your body.

SLOW DOWN: BE STILL AND KNOW

Stillness may not be the first thing that comes to mind when you think, *I need to lose some weight.* You probably expect to do lots of moving, sweating, and heavy breathing while relying on mental willpower and muscle flexing. Most likely you've tried this approach before. Maybe it even worked for a while, but it probably didn't last. This time, do it God's way—which tends to be the opposite of ours.

> The flesh desires what is contrary to the Spirit, and the Spirit what is contrary to the flesh. They are in conflict with each other, so that you are not to do whatever you want. But if you are led by the Spirit, you are not under the law.
>
> GALATIANS 5:17-18

The flesh accuses, pushes, prods, and pinches. The Spirit, who is stronger than any mental or physical muscle, does not. Scripture pictures Him as a dove—gentle and quiet.

Like Elijah, who did not encounter God in a strong wind, earthquake, or fire but in a gentle whisper (see 1 Kings 19:9-12), we will find the Spirit's strong but gentle presence in the secret and quiet places of our own hearts. To head out into the world without being intentionally wired into His voice and hooked up to His strength is a foolish waste of time. Learning to be still and meditate on the goodness of God teaches us to trust that God is active on our behalf. If we want to burn some serious calories, we must get serious about learning to be still.

A Kingdom wellness plan should include time for us to slow down so we can let the Holy Spirit come and create space between us and whatever is weighing us down. When we are still, we have time to learn proper alignment. That's why my favorite part of any fitness class is the cooldown: a time to lengthen tight muscles, lower the heart rate, and obtain good posture through intentional alignment. Over the years, I have noticed that mainstream fitness classes are shortening the cooldown to allow more time for the calorie burn. That's a shame, if you ask me. During the cooldown, we become aware of our thoughts and feelings and how they connect with our bodies.

As a fitness professional for more than twenty-five years, I have found significant benefits in practicing a form of yoga, which also teaches us to be still. The physical postures bring many benefits to my body—such as better blood flow and flexibility—all as I am meditating on God's Word in my mind and the love of Jesus in my heart.

When it comes to yoga, I am simply taking back what the enemy has stolen. Let me explain. Just because Hindus were the first to discover this good thing (the design of our physical bodies) and yoked it to a false god doesn't mean we have to lose it. Instead, I am taking back the postures that work for the body and yoking them to Jesus, who is the King of my heart. I call this "eating the meat and throwing out the bones." I throw out anything related to false worship (the bones), while I bring my whole body to "live and move and have [my] being" (Acts 17:28) in Him (the meat).

By slowing down, stretching, and taking time to decompress our minds and our muscles, we become more fit to move in love, and we avoid the chronic pain that comes from trying to complete a rigorous workout and hurriedly get on with our lives. As much as we push ourselves to do hard, sweaty things, we must also be willing to slow down and do kind and gentle things for our bodies.

This week, take time to lengthen and stretch your muscles while being intentional about breathing. You can start by practicing this for five to ten minutes a day. One idea: Wrap up your quiet time by sitting tall in your chair, in silence, breathing for five to ten counts in and out. As you are seated, fold forward and touch your toes as you continue to breathe. Let the breath be the sound track that supports the silence and makes you comfortable with it. You are training for godliness! God much prefers to whisper than to shout. Let Him.

You're also invited to check out RevWell TV to find "flexibility for your body and Jesus for your heart" workouts. Visit www.revelationwellness.org/workout-plans/revwell-tv/.

Be still and know!

MEDITATION

Meditation is not a New Age philosophy; instead, the New Age movement stole something that belonged to God, and He wants it back.

After all, Moses commanded Joshua, his successor, to "keep this Book of the Law always on your lips; meditate on it day and night, so that you may be careful to do everything written in it. Then you will be prosperous and successful" (Joshua 1:8).

Probably nobody was better versed in the discipline of meditation than King David. Whether running from salty King Saul or sitting on his royal throne, David knew that his strength came from God's promises, and he wasn't about to be shaken:

I meditate on your precepts and consider your ways.

PSALM 119:15

My eyes stay open through the watches of the night, that I may meditate on your promises.

PSALM 119:148

I will consider all your works and meditate on all your mighty deeds.

PSALM 77:12

Meditation is different from prayer in that, rather than talking to God, we simply consider the things of God. Prayer is conversation; meditation is contemplation. It allows the mind to wonder about, think about, chew on, and digest the things of God, while prayer petitions God to do something or to help us with something. Don't get me wrong; God invites us to petition Him and pursue Him for a breakthrough. But often our best protection against anything that threatens to kill, steal from, and destroy us comes from remembering, considering, and wondering about the goodness of God.

Meditation may feel risky because there are no rules. Through the psalmist, God tells us simply to "be still, and know that I am God" (Psalm 46:10). Meditation is more about delighting yourself in the Lord and being the object of His affection than waiting for a pep talk. Because it's so free flowing, if given a choice, our minds may drift away, or we may even find other things (like finally cleaning out that hallway closet) that seem more urgent than considering and delighting in the love of God. The enemy will try to use such distractions to divide our minds. The cunning one always carries a crowbar with him, and few things pry us from oneness with God more effectively than distractions. But when we pray and meditate, we draw near to God and the enemy must flee. He cannot stay on holy ground.

This week, look for opportunities to meditate. Maybe you will sit with God right after your prayer time. Or maybe you will decide to meditate instead of running to the break room for a doughnut when you get stressed at work. All you need to do is close your office door or head to a bathroom stall where you can sit and breathe and be the object of God's affection. Pull up a Bible passage on your smart phone and read until a word or a verse jumps out at you; then sit with it and breathe deeply until you encounter a greater peace, hope, or faith. Just think how much struggle we could avoid if we purposefully took time to breathe and consider the love of God. Talk about a violent act against the kingdom of darkness! You might also set up a place at home that is your sanctuary. This could be the secret place you go to "be still and know" when you are tempted to wring your hands and worry.

Wherever and however you choose to meditate, be intentional. Stay engaged with your breath and body, but not so much that they steal your focus from considering God and His Word. Holding a posture or connecting with your breath will help you maintain the proper balance between activity and passivity.

We must be willing to allow God to search us, look inside us, and expose anything that divides us from Him. We want Him to diagnose our hardness-of-heart disease. Meditation is like spiritual medication—it aids in the overall process of rehabbing our hearts and setting them free.

Some days you might be dry, feeling no motivation to draw near to God. On those days, meditation may come simply in the form of taking a moment to be still and let the dove, the Holy Spirit, rest on you. You might listen to some worship music or to the sound of silence. There are no rules. There are no time minimums and maximums. The only rule is not to fall into the trap of rating yourself on your ability to be attentive. Do not become a spiritual Pharisee who sets rules about how, where, and why to connect with God. Be open to the Holy Spirit's prompting to pray and ponder.

RENEW

With All Your Soul

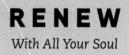

For study and application this week, take a deeper look at Romans 7:7-25. Read through this passage very slowly, chewing on the words and meditating on each verse. Ask the Lord to reveal truth to you bite by bite before reflecting on the following questions:

1. According to verses 7-12, how do we know we are sinning? When it comes to your health and well-being, where are you most likely to fall into sin?

2. Once we know the law, why is it that sin springs to life, causing us death? (See verses 9-11.)

3. What does God want for your health and well-being? How does Satan seek to destroy that plan in your mind?

4. Read Romans 7:13. What did Paul mean when he wrote, "Did the law, which is good, cause my death? Of course not! Sin used what was good to bring about my condemnation to death" (NLT)?

5. Reflect back upon these past four weeks. Are you beginning to see God bring about good changes in you by helping you kill any bad habits? If so, explain.

6. After reading verses 17-20, explain in your own words how you see the "battle" in your life as it pertains to you and your health and wholeness for God.

7. Read verses 21-23, where we are reminded that, even though we want to do good and delight in God's law in our inner beings, there is still another law at work. What law is that?

8. In verses 24-25, what emotions does Paul communicate? How does he describe his actions? Who, and only who, will rescue him (and us) from this body of death?

9. Read Romans 8:1-17. Verses 1-4 tell us there is no condemnation for us who are in Christ Jesus. Instead, what law sets us free from the law of sin and death? According to verse 3, what did God do to help us in our weakness with the law? What was the point of God sending Jesus in the flesh?

10. According to verses 5-6, what must we do to live in the law of the Spirit? And what do we receive when we live according to the Spirit and not the flesh?

God,

Thank You for saving me. Thank You for always thinking of me. I now ask for more of Your mind. Fill me with Your thoughts. I know the war that ensues inside me will not be won until I lay down the weapons of this world and put on my spiritual armor of salvation, righteousness, truth, and peace. Help me to raise my shield of faith to deflect the fiery darts of the enemy who hates to see me healthy, whole, and free. Help me wield the sword of Your Word, which is sharp enough to destroy anything that comes against me, and which removes my diseased thoughts. In Jesus' name, I take back all the stolen territory of my mind and mark it "Occupied by God." Fill my mind with more of Your truth and love.

✝ Amen.

RELATE

With All Your Mind and Strength

The following questions are designed to help you apply all you've learned this week to your fitness journey. Get with your accountability partner or small group and work honestly through these questions. Consider journaling your answers with God before sharing with your partner or group.

1. What are some common mind tricks the enemy likes to play on you? What happens when you fall for his tricks?

2. How often do you renew your mind? In addition to studying the Word, what could you do to renew your mind?

3. How comfortable are you with the idea of being still and pondering God and His Word? In our fast-paced world, what small step can you take to build some quiet into your schedule this week?

4. Share about a time in your life when you battled a lie and were able to hang on to the truth and win the battle.

RECIPROCATE

Finding the Bold in Her Soul

by Mariana Herrera Montaño,
Revelation Wellness Instructor

I am a volunteer instructor of Revelation Wellness fitness classes in an elementary school in Matamoros, Tamaulipas, in Mexico, for children with special needs. The classes are part of a program called CAM, and each of the kids who participate has at least one disability. When I began to volunteer there, my prayer was that God would use all that He had done in me so far to serve these children well. The truth is that I have learned much more about God through these children than I have taught them.

I know there is nothing I can do to be more loved by God. But the heart of God is that we love others as He first loved us. All of these special-needs children have struggled with their own physical conditions. They've experienced many painful moments, and many of their families live in poverty. In addition, they suffer the fear and insecurity of living in a region troubled by violence and drug trafficking. My desire is that they come to know that the love and grace of God can break any chain of bondage.

Lily is a beautiful twelve-year-old girl in the CAM program. Her mother abandoned her, and Lily was removed from her family because she was being abused. She has been diagnosed with a few mental disabilities. Lily is a very affectionate girl. When she sees me coming into the classroom, she runs to me and jumps with joy. Then she hugs and kisses me. She always says, "Teacher, I want to dance. What will we do in class today?" She tells me she loves me.

Through her, I have learned that God gives great wisdom to the humble. One day we were doing an activity called Bold in the Soul, where the kids are asked to write on their arm something that they believe God says about them. Lily asked me to write "Jesus." She told me, "Jesus is the bold in my soul 'cause He really loves me and makes me smart. He is my great love."

I am blessed to work with Lily and the other children. They are treasures to my heart. Every single child has a story to tell, and I experience the love of God each time I am with them.

ATTEND TO MATTERS OF THE HEART

I pray that you, being rooted and established in love, may have power, together with all the Lord's holy people, to grasp how wide and long and high and deep is the love of Christ, and to know this love that surpasses knowledge—that you may be filled to the measure of all the fullness of God.

EPHESIANS 3:17-19

I'm a recovering love-aholic. When I was young, I believed the lie that the love of a man would make me whole. I embraced the fairy tale that one day Prince Charming would sweep me off my feet. I loved watching romantic movies and daydreamed about having an elaborate wedding . . . followed by an uninterrupted happily ever after. Since everyone I knew seemed to want this, too, I never stopped to think that my quest for love had become an addiction.

I grew up in a home where more obvious addictions like alcohol abuse and adultery were present but not dealt with. And although my parents never separated or divorced, I didn't feel truly loved or safe growing up. I don't blame my parents for this feeling. I knew in my head they loved me, but my heart could never rest in this truth.

The enemy of our souls also used the addictions in my family to try to destroy the love between us. He went to work planting seeds of doubt and fear in my heart, hoping they would grow up twisted and stuck in the roots of lies. After all, love is a foundational and formative need, and if it isn't met, it grows into an insatiable want. And that is what happened. I didn't realize that the love I was looking for wasn't about warm feelings and romantic kisses but about the need to know I was safe, truly known, chosen, and accepted. As a result, I looked for love in all the wrong places.

After years of chasing love and then wondering why my husband didn't love me better, I finally understood the true condition of my own heart: No man would ever meet my desperate need for love and approval because God had created me to find my satisfaction in Him alone—the giver of all good gifts. Yet my sin separated me from God, and someone needed to pay the price so that breach could be mended. The great news I discovered was this—Jesus had willingly come to earth to take the punishment of sin upon Himself, dying a brutal death so that all who believe in this perfect love will have a restored relationship with their heavenly Father. Talk about limitless and relentless love! No matter how often we fall short, He never stops loving His kids.

Because God made us in His image, we are also meant to freely receive and give love. When a religious scholar asked Jesus what the most important commandment was, He replied, "Love the Lord your God with all your heart and with all your soul and with all your mind and with all your strength" (Mark 12:30). *All* means all—totally and completely.

If you are looking for complete transformation and lasting change, you must address the *whole* person. This is why "holistic medicine" has made such a name for itself in the past twenty years. People tire of treating symptoms while ignoring the causes of problems. *The Wellness Revelation* is all about moving you closer to the authentic person you were created to be. Let me assure you that while it does not come easily and brings some discomfort, what God wants to give you in exchange will not disappoint. He wants to give you a new heart as you learn to love Him completely.

What a high call! We are instructed to love God not just when we feel like it, but even when we don't. Unwilling hearts partnered with unrenewed minds keep people fragmented, compartmentalized, and separated from their best selves—running around getting their animalistic urges met in the moment instead of training for the higher prize of a life lived in right standing with God and filled with peace and joy.

Last week, we addressed the things that affect our minds. This week, let's dive deeper into matters of the heart. First, we need to remember that we were created in the image of a loving God and hardwired for emotional and relational connection. God designed man and woman so that we would need Him. Our feelings are given to us by God to draw us closer to Himself, the One who is Love and the author of feelings. Because He wastes nothing, He is able to make even the negative feelings work for our good (see Romans 8:28).

Remember to use your **Moving Forward Journal** this week to track your food and water intake, as well as to remain focused on this week's Scripture verse. You can download a copy at www.revelationwellness.org/book/workout or photocopy the template on page 239.

Why, then, is heart transformation so difficult?

When we receive bad news or have a negative thought, we are supposed to look for immediate comfort. The issue is not *if* we will feel bad; it's *what* we will do when we feel bad. Will we run our hearts to the pantry for comfort, or to God, our Comforter? At some point, we have all been hurt, cheated, deceived, rejected, or ridiculed by other people who have also been wounded. While the scars of physical wounds are more obvious, whenever we believe the wrong words and messages of others, we are scarred on the inside as well. Our fractured hearts make it harder for us to trust and focus on God so that we can receive His love and live as people set apart for His good and great things.

When neglected, these spiritual wounds become infected and spread. Satan, the father of all lies, hopes we get so spiritually sick that he can kill us and destroy the legacy God wants to give us. He offers the bait of dark and shameful places where we find momentary relief but no freedom. While drugs and alcohol are the most obvious forms of self-medication, he will encourage our tendencies to use food, shopping, work, achievement, celebrity, media, and romantic love to numb the pain as well. At that point, our calloused hearts become desensitized to God, and we become fit for Satan's purposes of bringing more hell to earth. The liar is not jealous for our worship; he's jealous of God. He doesn't care where we go for comfort, as long as it's not to God.

In addition to the hurt inflicted upon us by others, our hearts are influenced by our fallen human nature, which says, *What's in it for me? Why should I choose to love when no one seems to love me back?* When we place expectations or rules on our love—in fact, wherever there are rules—there is loss of freedom. Wherever rules expand, freedom contracts. Don't misunderstand me; rules designed to protect our freedom are good. A sense of right and wrong is necessary for a well-lived life. Abuse, for instance, should never be tolerated in the name of love. Yet there is one place where there are no rules, and that is in the giving of love—pure love, because we have been loved.

It's not easy to rest in the love of God. Over the years, I developed a serious "heart infection." I knew something was wrong when I was proclaiming my faith verbally but was continually frustrated, burned out, and exhausted internally. Though my heart was full of zeal for the Lord, my mind kept playing old tapes that got in the way of my ability to love. I was proclaiming God's endless love, while in my marriage, I wanted to quit. In the ministry, I wanted to quit. I even wanted to quit some of the friendships I never thought would fail. My heart was flatlining. Over and over I wanted to quit.

And yet this feeling of frustration was my lifesaver—it confirmed that something was off. In my exhaustion, I asked God to fix me! God, the Good Surgeon, faithfully examined my heart and pointed out the cause of my spiritual heart disease. The culprit was expectations—first of God, and then of other people. As I grew, the Lord showed me the deeper issues of my heart—that my unhealthy expectations of others developed because of my past hurts.

Sometimes even believers in Christ wonder where God has gone or if He even exists. After all, He isn't meeting our expectations. In our search for answers, we spot the sign in the road between our hearts and our minds that reads, "God is not good." So we jump on the first bus out of town, failing to see the road sign that says Rebel Road. This road is full of pleasures and attractions guaranteed to amuse us and relieve our pain. Often we turn to these false functional saviors for some relief.

Because it's so easy to take the detour onto Rebel Road and fall into a ditch, we need continual realignment checks all day long. We need to hear the Father say, "Eyes up here" in the moments we feel sucker punched by the inner critic who calls us fat because our pants don't fit or when our self-esteem deflates because we didn't get the compliment we were looking for. God knows that apart from a checkup from the neck up—a realignment of our minds—we will respond in fear and run from Him.

And even when we have veered off onto Rebel Road, we will eventually fall down and wave a white flag in surrender. Stuck somewhere in a dark alley of the soul, in an unsearched place between heart and mind, we are likely to run out of rebellious steam. We feel abandoned and confused, so we cry out for God's mercy. And God comes. His presence enters the darkness and reminds us that we are never without Him and His hope. Why did we rush off so quickly? Where did we go?

We must remember that nowhere in God's greatest commandment does He say, "Love God with all your heart, mind, and soul, and everything will go perfectly for you." God desires that we love Him out of our own free will, not in exchange for what He will do for us or what He can give us. He also desires that we love others in the same way He loves us. We must remember that, just as Christ loved us sacrificially, He is not commanding us to love for our own satisfaction and gratification, but so that we may give and receive life through our love for others.

Placing expectations on people is the quickest way to dash our hopes. People will fail us, our circumstances will fail us, but our God never will. He came to bind up the brokenhearted, proclaim good news, provide freedom for the captives, and release the prisoners from darkness (see Isaiah 61:1). I had to learn to set aside all my expectations other than the expectation—no, the never-failing truth—that God will remain good and faithful. He will do what He says He will do. And while I am waiting for Him to do it, I can strengthen myself in the joy of the Lord, which is my strength (see Nehemiah 8:10).

God's love is not a commodity. You cannot trade and exchange God's love. Why would we want to exchange gold for paper, anyway? You cannot leverage yourself against the love of God. He is not looking for business partners. He's looking for a family: children who are willing to go into the family business of transforming the world through His love and truth, which sets hearts free.

God's love never quits. His love is inexhaustible and continues to flow to those who love Him—and even to those who don't. Just like a good father, He doesn't love you because you obey Him, but He will continue to love you until you want to obey Him! Until pleasing His heart makes your heart whole, He will keep loving you.

We know that weight loss is not rocket science. Eat less, move more. That would work great—if we were machines designed simply to take in and output data. However, our feelings often drive us to the pantry rather than into the presence of God. When we find ourselves force-feeding our feelings with food, or restricting food in order to gain some sense of control, know this: God is not crossing His arms and tapping His foot, shaming us with a "You should know better." His love is patient. His love is kind (see 1 Corinthians 13:4). God's love doesn't "should" on us. He knows our pain. He knows why we turn back to other sources of comfort rather than Him. Our Father always takes us back and gives us a "love makeover." He restores our hope and renews our faith. At our request, He gives us back His treasure map, showing us the way to seek and find what will really give us rest—His love. He resets our hearts' compasses and says, "If you start to feel lost again, point this toward home." He then aligns our willing hearts, minds, souls, and bodies with His will for our lives. In His presence our hearts are healed and made whole.

Be aware, however, that we will feel His absence again. It will come when things don't go the way we expect—in times of trials that test our faith. And when that disappointment comes, what will we do?

When it feels as if God has left us, it's decision time. We must remember the roads we have traveled, remember where we have been and what God has done. We have already been down Rebel Road, and we know where that leads. This time, if we don't panic and don't respond in fear, if we take the time to breathe and recall and recite truth, we will hear God whisper, "Do not move! Wait here. I'm coming. Start declaring how faithful I am, and your fear will flee."

We are saved by grace, through faith. Whenever and wherever we declare faith, grace shows up to do the work of heaven on earth through us, and we are equipped to think, feel, and act in step with the Kingdom.

When you wonder if God has pulled away, remain still. Trust that God is near even in the stillness and silence. Above all else, remember He loves you, even when you can't feel Him. His love never quits!

FUELED BY GRACE

Love is God's motive, but grace is His fuel. Excuse me while I get a little fired up . . . but I think we often misunderstand grace. We throw the word around like a dirty, wet mop that we pull out to clean up our messes. "Oh, you did that again?" we say. "Don't worry. Give yourself grace." No sir . . . this is not grace at all.

As sinners, we receive mercy from God first:

> God, being rich in mercy, because of the great love with which he loved us, even when we were dead in our trespasses, made us alive together with Christ—by grace you have been saved.
>
> EPHESIANS 2:4-5, ESV

Mercy is not giving people what they deserve. Grace is giving people what they need.

When I was a kid, my brother and I loved to leg wrestle. We would lie on our backs, and one of us would shout, "I declare a leg war!" The war proceedings would begin with a "One, two, three, four" as we swung our legs back and forth in rhythm with the count. Considering my four-foot frame and his five-foot frame, guess who would usually win? Within thirty seconds of my brother pinning my little Chihuahua leg behind my back, I would gruffly shout the magic word, "Mercy!" Though my brother was in the position to give me a hamstring pull, he never hurt me. This is mercy.

When we sin, we deserve separation from God, ourselves, and others. But God refuses to give us what we deserve. That is mercy. Then God, being rich in mercy, goes even further and gives us what we need—kindness and the reminder of who we are because we are so greatly loved!

We are a new creation, the chosen children of God, and agents of change for the world. Because of what Christ did on the cross, not only does God in His mercy *not* give us what we deserve, He gives us Himself, His love, and our identities as royal heirs. That's grace—God's undeserved gift to us, which is immeasurably more than we can ask or imagine (see Ephesians 3:20)! Grace cannot be earned, but it must be received and cared for so that our identities are not stolen from us again.

Grace is not permission to live according to the flesh but power to live by the Spirit. Like God's love, it never quits! It enables us to live in step with God's Spirit and to do what we never thought we could. Our "who" (our identity) will be rightly connected to our "do" (what we do and how we do it).

Grace is not a backup plan for when we fall short and need a cleanup on aisle ten. Grace is *the* plan! God's grace, just like His love, is available to anyone in an unending supply. Just call on His name. If you lack the fuel, the ability to say no to the cravings of your flesh and yes to the things of God, just ask for His grace. As the apostle Paul wrote, "My God will meet all your needs according to the riches of his glory in Christ Jesus" (Philippians 4:19).

If you feel discouraged by what I am saying because you thought you were living under grace but getting nowhere, please don't fear. This is an exciting time for you! Mercy keeps the believer on heaven's life support, while grace gives the believer life to the full!

Now God wants to wreck you with His love. He wants to give you a fresh revelation of just how loved you are. Once you step into His "unforced rhythms of grace" (Matthew 11:29, MSG), your transformation is sure to begin. But it

GRACE IS NOT PERMISSION TO LIVE ACCORDING TO THE FLESH BUT POWER TO LIVE BY THE SPIRIT.

will continually cost you your old ways of thinking and feeling—your more comfortable ways of living. Are you ready for an upgrade?

Try to envision God's love as a fountain that flows eternally and abundantly. He can't help but give and give and give. You are the vessel that God desires to continually fill. Instead of obsessing over how you are going to fill your belly, let God fill your heart. He wants your heart to be full and your needs to be met so that you will be able to help meet the needs of others. His love is meant to fill you first, then overflow to others. This is what Jesus had in mind when He said, "I have come that they may have life, and have it to the full" (John 10:10).

Loving God

Before Jesus came and identified "the greatest commandment," God had given His people the Ten Commandments—the one and only Top Ten List.

Have you ever noticed books, magazines, radio spots, or news/talk shows that want to break solutions down into "ten easy steps"? God knows that people respond to rules and guidelines in numeric form. Allow me to paraphrase these commandments:

God is the only God!

Have no idols or false gods (e.g., food, fitness, drugs, sex, social media, money, success—things that get in the way of God).

Do not speak about God without respect for who He is.

Keep a day of rest. You're kind of cranky when you don't. And nobody's drawn to a cranky Christian.

Honor your parents even when they don't do anything worth honoring. They gave you life. That is to be honored.

Don't kill anyone. And remember your words have the ability to kill hope, visions, and dreams or to give life to hope, visions, and dreams.

Don't have sex outside of marriage. Sex is a physical representation of a covenant love between God and humanity. Save sex for the life promise met in marriage. Doing so will keep your heart from breaking over and over again.

Don't take anything that is not yours.

Don't bend the truth. It only gives way to lies.

Don't long for people, power, or possessions that belong to someone else.

These are God's simple rules for well-being. Simple, yes, but not easy. Our flesh gets in the way, either to persuade us to give in to momentary pleasures or to point out that we will never measure up. There's nothing wrong with wanting to please God with our actions, but we should never make impressing God more important than pressing into God.

Christ came to do what we could not—fulfill the law perfectly. He also left us the gift of the Holy Spirit, who equips us to do what our rule-following forefathers never could—live on good terms with God and rest in His love. We went from ten rules chiseled in stone to God alive in us! We are not worthy of such a thing, which is why we clothe ourselves in humility.

We will always need more grace and love flowing in and out of our lives. When you are tempted to sin, look for grace and look for love. They flow in the opposite direction of the world, so their current can initially be hard to find. Feel for the resistance. It's there that the Kingdom of God is found within you.

Loving Yourself

One of the most overlooked aspects of a powerful Christian love, a pure God-love, is the realization that you are called to love yourself well. In God's eyes, you are endlessly loved and relentlessly pursued. He won't stop—can't stop—loving you!

How good are you at loving yourself? I am going to challenge you with a tough question: If you love God and love yourself, why do you eat yourself into a state of physical weakness? Or malnourish yourself out of fear of getting fat?

Why do you overwork yourself into a state of anxiety, stress, and high blood pressure? Or smoke cigarettes that you know are killing you?

When we lose sight of God's love for us, the enemy will try to get us to sabotage ourselves by turning to idols for comfort. If that doesn't work, he will tempt us to embrace ourselves as idols. Satan directs our eyes toward earthly pleasures and tempts us to tell ourselves, "I deserve this," rather than remembering that God's love is absolute and undeserved. Distorted forms of self-love lead to pride and harden our hearts toward the divine nature and will of God.

I have seen the "me" of this world. Oh, friends, she isn't pretty. On the outside, she looks quite put together, but on the inside, she's a wreck. She is afraid of being rejected, not chosen, and not enough. She will do whatever she needs to do to be loved, jumping through all the cosmetic beauty hoops in an effort to live up to today's definition of a "real" woman. She is following a current that flows directly opposite to God's "unforced rhythms of grace."

Thankfully, God searches my heart, and He is keenly aware of the battleground in my mind. When I cry out to Him, He shows up ready to rescue and save. He declares "Peace, be still" to the storm in my mind (see Mark 4:39, NKJV).

Often, I need to be reminded of who I am in God's eyes. I need to remember that He really likes me and enjoys me—that He is jealous for my time and affection. It is in my alone time, away from all my roles as a wife, mother, daughter, and leader, that I am reminded of the real me, who doesn't have to do anything to satisfy God. It pleases Him to see me enjoying Him. The real me, the best me, is the girl who enjoys being with and hearing from her heavenly Dad. This is why the practice of retreating, getting away with God, even if it is just for five minutes, is important to sustaining the wellness revival in our souls.

When God's Son died on the cross for you and me, He threw Himself over us to cover our mess—our guilt and shame—because love covers a multitude of sins (see 1 Peter 4:8). Once we confess that Jesus is our Savior, God the Father sees Christ covering us, making us complete, even when we are not yet whole.

Thankfully, as Christ followers we have been given access to the Holy Spirit, who always stands ready to remind us of God's love and to equip us to act from that pure love. We must choose to receive and rest in that love so that when the storms come, we will remember and declare who is fighting for us!

When we extend to ourselves the same grace that He extends to us on a daily basis, it makes our heavenly Dad beam. Wherever you see kindness, you see grace in action—grace showing off so the face of God might be seen.

Who would you be if you decided to live under this one charge? "Today I will be kind. I will speak only kind words about myself and others. I will entertain only kind thoughts about myself and others. I will eat food that is kind to my body. I will go to the gym and move my body as an act of kindness. I am kind because my King is kind."

Kindness is good medicine for our hearts. After all, God's kindness leads us toward repentance (see Romans 2:4). And God's kind of people are kind.

How fun would it be if the people of God became so healthy and whole from the inside out that when people began to wonder what had changed for us, we could reply, "I am on the kindness diet! I have learned to be kind to myself because God is always so kind to me." Come on, church. Let's be like that! God's love would surely flow from us to others then!

Loving Others

I always find it absurd that God chooses to partner with broken people to show His love to the world. If we choose not to value ourselves, be kind to ourselves, and have a healthy and whole love for ourselves, how will the world ever experience God's pure love through us? The second greatest commandment is "Love your neighbor as yourself" (Mark 12:31).

Jesus' ministry was based on one primary work: love. Think about it. God Himself put on a suit of flesh and blood. He could have come down and gotten on a cosmic PA system and ordered, "All of you, worship Me!" Then He could have gone right back to heaven. Instead, God came down and put His hands in the dirt. He humbled Himself and put Himself side by side with those who were broken, abused, neglected, and impoverished as well as with the clean-cut, got-it-all-together, hard-hearted religious folk. All these people were His people. He was sent to heal them, bind up their wounds, and love them. When we're honest, we recognize that "they" are us.

When God's love flows through our hearts, we are healthy and whole. We can then produce good fruit that nourishes others. When we desire to reflect the beauty of Christ in our hearts and our minds, we effectively bear fruit from our hearts first; then our hands will give that fruit away.

Galatians 5:22-23 tells us what this fruit looks like: "The fruit of the Spirit is love, joy, peace, forbearance, kindness, goodness, faithfulness, gentleness and self-control. Against such things there is no law." Paul is speaking of godly traits, the embodiment of God's character that is ours for the asking. When we possess these virtues, we are no longer slaves to the law but to Jesus Christ, who sets us free!

In my backyard, I have countless citrus trees. They produce more grapefruit and oranges each year than I can use. It seems a shame that I can't keep up with their bounty or fully appreciate their supply when they are doing what God created them to do! I don't do anything to encourage or nourish the trees to grow or reproduce; they just do. As long as their root systems are not messed with, those trees will continue to produce lots of fruit even after I have passed on. It's quite a marvel to think that good seed, buried and dead, grew into a grove of trees and that those trees will continue to produce fruit until they are uprooted or Christ returns—whichever comes first.

God is calling us to be lavish givers just like those trees in my backyard. When we remain rooted in Him and His love, we can't help but produce more because that is who we are and what we do. Even if my husband and children don't sing my praises each week for doing laundry, cooking meals, running errands, and tending to a growing ministry, I will continue to bear fruit. If fruit falls from my branches and no one is around to eat it, I am no less of a fruit tree. A fruit tree is a fruit tree because it produces fruit, not because somebody eats the fruit.

Love, joy, peace, forbearance, kindness, goodness, faithfulness, gentleness, and self-control do not start and stop with us. These character traits change us and compel us "to act justly and to love mercy and to walk humbly with [our] God" (Micah 6:8). When we see this fruit in our lives, we know that God's love has indeed changed us from the inside out.

GOD'S WELLNESS PLAN

By the grace of God's Word and His love, may you get this: God wants to heal your heart so that you may have deeper faith for wholehearted living and a fuller life. He wants you to be holy (producing the fruit of the Spirit) and whole (healthy in heart, mind, and body) so that you will be fully alive, a living testimony to God's goodness and faithfulness. This is God's wellness plan for all humankind.

We must live well because we can't help our neighbors if we can't help ourselves. God's love does not, cannot, and will not stop with us. Before Jesus comes back, we point others to God's hope. Will we make the difference in a hurting world by turning away from those familiar and comfortable habits that ensnare us? If we give God our hearts *and* our bodies, we will be able to help others break free from their own traps.

Ask God to deliver you from the chains and whispered deceptions that keep you from bearing fruit. Jesus did not die so that those deceptions would bury you alive and leave you feeling overwhelmed, paralyzed, and numb. When God's love displaces the lies in your heart, something amazing happens—you receive an overflow that is meant to be poured out on others. Next time you walk into a room, walk in completely confident in who you are because of whose you are. Make a decision to enter every situation as a royal son or daughter who has all the resources of heaven. Freely sow seeds of love, and name what is excellent in people or situations, even if they look hopeless.

If you have exhausted your good seed, go back to your secret place where you meet with the Voice of Love. He will refill you; He never runs out of seed!

Meditate on this truth: *God, my Father, really, really, really loves me. He loves me because He loves me because He loves me. He won't change His mind about me. The way He loves me is how He loves others. He is counting me worthy to love like Him, right here, right now.*

Love refuses human-imposed rules; it resists charts, graphs, and measuring tools. Love does not demand this for that. Love moves and flows freely from God to us to others and back again. God is love. And His love is the ultimate divine weight-loss plan—lifting the self-hatred, pride, and fear that burden us.

RESPOND

With All Your Heart

Continue to respond to God's love and truth for you through the movement of your body using this week's training plan. See page 240 to access the Wellness Revelation Workout Calendar for the link to each day's workout video.

THE BUTTERFLY—FREEDOM

After a short time of struggle, every caterpillar emerges from the dark into the light, transformed into a glorious butterfly. The creature that once slowly but faithfully scooted across the dirt now takes its maiden voyage with wings.

If you are still in the cocoon you entered in week 3, you are now invited to emerge and give your wings a try. Three weeks is a healthy amount of time to retrain your taste buds to prefer new flavors and to create new habits for your mind. If you have abstained from soda, candy, and other sugary foods, you may find a sip or bite of your former favorite now tastes offensively strong. However, you may still find those foods familiar and comforting. Continue to look for new flavors and for foods packed with nutrition.

You are now in a new and exciting phase, similar to that of a butterfly that has broken free from the cocoon to explore the world from a new perspective. The difference is that you have developed godly self-discipline. Allow me to offer some guidelines you can use as guardrails to keep you from driving into the ditches of pride and unbelief, either neglecting or obsessing about your body. Each one of these guidelines is practical and can be used by anyone desiring to live healthy and whole—whether or not you're just exiting a cocoon.

Before you decide whether to follow any of these guidelines, pray and ask the Father if it is something He wants you to do at this time.

YOUR BODY

Food

One day a week, consider allowing yourself some food freedom. This makes room for birthday parties, weddings, and other special occasions that are part of a good and godly life. Since you are learning "love obedience" by being sensitive to the Spirit and intentional about how much, when, and what types of food you eat, this one day a week will not master you. On this day, you are the master of food, enjoying food without allowing it to consume you. This one day a week will keep you from becoming the food police—living under rules and regulations and calling it freedom. It will also help you identify the foods that just don't work for you anymore, so you can decide what to abstain from and when. Just like a butterfly, we seek freedom as our goal!

As you move through this day of freedom, be sure to enjoy the flavors, smells, and textures of your food, taking your time and being present so you can savor the moment and remember it is not about the food. Rich foods are to be enjoyed as a gift from God, who has richly blessed us with all things. A good meal is meant to point us toward a good God!

Please don't interpret this as a challenge to see how much food you can ingest in one day. You're too sober and smart for that kind of nonsense! When it becomes about you and your wants, you may begin to fall down a slippery slope. Don't panic. Stay sober, call on Jesus' name, and watch for the grace that will equip you to move toward the Spirit. Get back in step with Him.

In addition to considering a weekly day of freedom, continue eating primarily high-octane fuel for food—fruits and vegetables, whole grains, nuts, seeds, clean meats, and healthy fat.

Continue exercising the "4S" of feeding your body when you eat:

Slow: Take the time to be present when it's time to eat.

Sufficient: Be thoughtful about how much goes on your plate.

Satisfied: Eat until you are satisfied, not stuffed. (Continue using the 1–5 hunger scale.)

Steady: Stay ahead of your hunger by eating steadily throughout the day.

Consider using your food journal when you know you are becoming mindless and going numb about what and when you are eating.

If you find that you are starting to sneak in extra food and it's not due to true hunger because of increased activity and muscle growth, take some time to pray. Get sober, get quiet, and ask God what's going on with you. If you feel as if you are losing your free self, a fast is in order (either a traditional food fast or an element fast). Go back to the Respond sections in weeks 2 and 3. Read and reset.

Drink

If you can have alcohol without alcohol having you, one to two glasses of alcohol per week can be appropriate. Of course, this does not apply if alcohol has been an idol or addiction in the past. If you know that alcohol can easily take you captive, numb your senses, impair your reasoning, and prevent you from making good choices, I think it is safe to say the Lord would like you to stay free of it. Keep it on the altar, and keep your hands off it. His love is more intoxicating!

Fitness

As you make fitness a regular part of your life, remember to:

- Move your body at least four days (and up to six days) a week for thirty minutes.
- Complete resistance training at least twice a week.

- Value the art of movement for movement's sake and stay away from the "all or nothing" principle. Remember that a ten-minute workout is better than nothing. Move your body as an act of worship before your God. Choose quality of movement over quantity of time. Whole people value moving well over moving more.
- Make time to stretch and breathe at least three to six times a week for at least five to ten minutes. Right after a workout is best. Use this time to center your heart in the Lord before heading out to tackle the day.
- Extend yourself grace and get back in step with the Spirit as soon as possible after missing one or more workouts.

YOUR SPIRIT

When you open yourself to the Spirit, He will work in the secret places, strengthening you with His love and equipping you to love yourself and others in a fruitful way. Be sure to:

- Study God's Word and apply it to your life as often as possible.
- Spend regular time, even if it's just two to five minutes a day, sitting in the presence of God and meditating on His love.
- Seek out a community of Christ followers who don't just help you feel better but help you get better.

If you find yourself wandering during this new season of freedom and feeling anxious, stuck, or less joy-filled or peaceful than you once were, consider whether the Spirit is inviting you to return to God through a traditional or element fast. Remember that fasting is not meant as a punishment or a ritual but as a time set aside for seeking and hearing from God and for breaking chains. It is never a diet.

Love Others

Freedom is never free. It has a price. Galatians 5:13 reminds us, "You, my brothers and sisters, were called to be free. But *do not use your freedom to indulge the flesh; rather, serve one another humbly in love*" (emphasis mine).

Back in the book's introduction, we talked about how as we become healthier and more whole, we can love others as we love God. When we give away the same things we ourselves need, God gives back to us in greater measure. Our bodies and lives will fall in line with the unforced rhythms of love and grace.

I bet God is calling you to spend some of yourself on someone in your life. Perhaps you've been withholding forgiveness from someone. Perhaps God keeps asking you to do something that you continually disqualify yourself from doing. When we obey God's promptings, we are living out wellness in the most powerful way. The world will tell you to hunker down and self-focus your way into healthy living. I am here to tell you that God's hands are always open, and He wants you to open your hands too!

This week I challenge you to take a risk, be intentional, and do something to give away love. Warning: If you give it away expecting something in return, you may be highly disappointed. Expectations are premeditated resentments. Exercise your God-given identity and power to freely give away what you need: *love!*

Pray about this. Ask God to provide you an opportunity to show real love in a conscious and deliberate way. I can promise that this will be more powerful if you step outside your comfort zone. Nothing new happens inside our comfort zones. Get comfortable being uncomfortable.

Love others even when it is *not* what you feel like doing. Or love impulsively because you see a need or can heal a hurt. God is always moving around us and asking us to participate in the dance, so dance!

Journal about your experience. I predict you may feel so alive, connected, and purposeful in this exercise that you will want to dance some more. Stay humble and show others the face of love.

RENEW

With All Your Soul

The Old Testament book of Deuteronomy records Moses' farewell address to the nation of Israel. In addition to urging them to follow the Lord's commands, Moses reminded the people of God's faithfulness and of His "mighty hand, his outstretched arm; the signs he performed and the things he did in the heart of Egypt" (11:2-3).

1. Describe a memorable time when God outstretched His mighty hand to you. Why would the God of the universe do such a thing?

2. Read Deuteronomy 11:8-9. How does this passage make clear that God cares about His people's well-being?

3. Taking into account any changes in your perspective on food and drink since beginning this study, what would you say "a land flowing with milk and honey" (verse 9) means for your life in this present day and culture?

4. Read verses 10-15. What do these verses say about God's love for His children? What does He long to give you? According to verse 13, what did God require from His people in order to give them all these good things? What might that look like in your own life?

5. In verses 14-15, God says, "I will send rain on your land in its season, both autumn and spring rains, so that you may gather in your grain, new wine and olive oil. I will provide grass in the fields for your cattle, and you will eat and be satisfied." The ending is especially powerful. Please fill in the blank: "I will provide grass in the fields for your cattle, and you will eat and be _____." What does this tell you about what God wants for you?

6. Read verse 16. How do you think it is connected to verse 15?

7. Why do you think God *must be* your sufficiency always? How has this truth become a reality for you as you've worked through the first six weeks?

8. Read 1 Corinthians 13:1-3. Summarize what Paul is telling us about this God quality called love.

9. In verses 4-8, Paul outlines the qualities that make up love. They are listed below. Next to each one, write a brief explanation showing how this particular godly trait connects to your health and wholeness physically and spiritually.

(Example) Patient: *Patience is hard for me. I am short fused and can feel this in my body when my heart feels anxious. I know that if I get ahead of God, I get exhausted trying to act in my own strength.*

Patient

Kind

Does not envy

Does not boast

Not proud

Does not dishonor others

Not self-seeking

Not easily angered

Keeps no record of wrongs

Rejoices with the truth

Protects

Trusts

Hopes

Perseveres

10. Consider how living without each trait affects your heart and mind. In addition, what common bodily responses do you notice when you do not love like this?

Dear Jesus,

I am Your child who needs Your love in order to know what love is. Help me, Lord, never to forget that it is because of Your great, uncontainable, and never-ending love that You decided to create everything, with me as one of the centerpieces of Your love. I desire to love You more because You love me more than anyone else does, and You know what is best for my life. Please take my heart of stone and return it to me as a heart of flesh. Because I know that Your love is the remedy for the world's pain, I desire to have more God-love so that I may give more God-love.
✛ Amen.

RELATE

With All Your Mind and Strength

The following questions are designed to help you apply all you've learned this week to your fitness journey. Get with your accountability partner or small group and work honestly through these questions. Consider journaling your answers with God before sharing with your partner or group.

1. When you are tempted, how does your body react physically? Please describe (e.g., you sweat, bite your lip, or feel your heart race). If you are not sure, pay attention to your response the next time you feel the urge to do something you know you shouldn't. Then record what you observe below.

2. How often have you sat with discomfort or pain during temptation this week? Were you able to sit with it until you found peace and resolution? If so, explain what that felt like.

3. What experiences, whether recently or in the past, illustrate God's love for you? If you can't think of anything, what might be preventing you from believing that God loves you personally and deeply?

4. Name at least one character trait you love about yourself. Name one physical characteristic you find most attractive about yourself.

5. What are the top three things you love most about God? What are three things that you think God loves most about you?

RECIPROCATE

Sam's Story

by Mimi Foster,
Revelation Wellness Instructor

S
am walked into my fitness class for teens on a cool fall evening. The eight-
week class was part of the nonprofit Love INC's midweek family program
that offered participants a number of classes and a free hot meal. Attendees
received points for being there, which they could spend on items in our "store."

Sam had a wild mop of curls and a scowl that was meant to intimidate anyone who got in his way. In that first class, I could tell that he wanted no part of
anything I was teaching. While everyone else goofed around and settled in, Sam
sat on a beanbag chair and said that he wasn't going to do anything. Before our
workout, I talked with the teens about the pressures they felt from social media.
Sam kept trying to disrupt the class, though he did follow the group outside
when we went to do some workouts with drumsticks, fitness props that enabled
us to move our bodies to the beat of the music. At the end of the night, I prayed
with the students and distributed their participation points. When I awarded
Sam full points, he gave me a funny look.

My assistant Mindy and I talked after class. We agreed that Sam had likely
been unsettled to find two new teachers when he walked into the room. (He
didn't have a lot of stability in his life.) We were determined to help him realize
that our class was a safe place and that he was loved.

The next week Sam came in wearing the same scowl. When it was time to
work out, he picked up the drumsticks, though he said he was not going to participate because his legs hurt from gym class. I told him that was fine and that
if he felt up to it, he could join in at any time. (Inside I was rejoicing because

he had expressed how he was feeling.) Afterward I took prayer requests, and Mindy and I prayed over them. Just before handing out participation points, we reminded the teens we were always there for them if they needed us.

Week 3 was pivotal in our relationship with Sam. During our discussion time, he told us how he felt about himself and talked about what was happening at school. He joined in with our workout, and a smile replaced his scowl!

In the following weeks, we watched God go to work in Sam's life. He took on a leadership role among the other students and asked how he could help Mindy and me. He even led the group in prayer a few times! We watched this boy find new life in Christ and gain some self-esteem in the process.

On the last night of class, we decided to send everyone home with positive words of affirmation. We wrote each person's name on a paper plate, passed the plates around, and asked the teens to write positive words about the person whose name was on the plate. Sam had so many wonderful things to say about his peers, and they filled his plate with just as many loving words. As we prayed and they all walked out the door, Mindy and I cried because of the huge impact the group had made on our lives. Sam in particular taught me that no matter what situation people are coming from, God can break through if I allow Him to soften up their hearts through my loving words and actions so they can trust again!

BE TRANSFORMED

If anyone is in Christ, the new creation has come:

The old has gone, the new is here!

2 CORINTHIANS 5:17

I'm a woman who was wrecked by the love of Jesus, and I didn't even see it coming.

I was once a woman who could tell you easily what was wrong, and it always had something to do with someone else: *If only [insert name] would [insert action] then I could [insert desired feeling, thought, or action].* I had built my life on the philosophy of me. I was stuck on me. And I was sick of me. Sin kept me from realizing that life is about making God the point of everything I do. And here's the crazy part: Once I made God the point of my life, He seemed to say, "Hey, everyone, this is My daughter; listen to her! She spends time with Me, so she knows some of My secrets—the ones you are running around like crazy trying to figure out."

God is using me in some of the same ways He used Jesus. And He wants to do the same with you.

To this day, when I am feeling stuck and lacking hope, faith, or the ability to love, I am pretty quick to realize that I am the problem because I have made myself the point. My love for God continues to tear down any monuments I build in honor of myself so that God can continue to build His temple in me.

I am not the woman I used to be.

My poor husband. Simon had no idea what he was getting when he married me. Six months after I gave my heart back to the Lord, I was noticeably changing. I stopped trying to make my husband my savior. Jesus had that position now. I remember a moment when I was getting ready to leave our house for church. Simon got right in front of me, put his hands firmly on my shoulders, looked me in the eyes, and said, "Now, you're not going to become some sort of Jesus freak, are you?" With great conviction and assurance, I smirked and said, "No way!"

At the time I didn't really understand that Jesus came not simply to save us, keep us safe, and get us home, but to return us to wholeness. God sent His one and only Son, Jesus, to save us from ourselves and to make us more and more like Him. God's love redeems and restores us to our original design. Through the frustrations of daily life and the pain of challenging circumstances, He transforms us into greater Christlikeness.

Friends, may I confess that my name is Alisa Keeton and today I am a bona fide Jesus freak. It's nice to meet you. I invite you to let God—not your spouse, your kids, your job, your body, your age, your ability, your talent, your gifting, or anything else—be your Savior. Let God love you and tell you who He created you to be. Then by the power of His love, He will enable you to become that person. You will lose your little old life in exchange for a new, exciting, not-dependent-upon-any-person-or-circumstance life!

If I'd been paying attention to the apostle Paul when Simon stopped me in our hallway, I might have seen it coming: "We were therefore buried with him through baptism into death in order that, just as Christ was raised from the dead through the glory of the Father, we too may live a new life" (Romans 6:4).

Back then I wasn't looking to die or to be baptized into death. I thought I could keep the love of God under control, but little did I know. I have been transformed by His love, and God wants to change you in the same way. Will you let Him?

One of my favorite parables is the one Jesus told about the man who finds a treasure hidden in a field. He is so excited that he hides it again and then goes and sells everything he has to buy that plot of land. Unfortunately, I think God gives the treasure of salvation—a free and forgiven life—to many Christians who bury their treasure but never buy the field. The whole point of buying the field is for us to take ownership of the land that comes with the treasure. If we just stick the treasure in our pockets like a rabbit's foot we covertly stroke three times for luck, we will miss out on being the people we could have become,

---

Remember to use your **Moving Forward Journal** this week to track your food and water intake, as well as to remain focused on this week's Scripture verse. You can download a copy at www.revelationwellness.org/book/workout or photocopy the template on page 239.

---

and we will shortchange everyone who could have benefited from us buying the field and going all in with our faith. Many believers may go to church, tithe, hang Scripture plaques in their homes, and enjoy a Bible study or memorize a key verse now and then. But inwardly they haven't given up everything to gain the treasure that is theirs in Christ. They are stuck in what I call a "salvation slump"—they know about God's love and power but continually try living from their own power and ability.

Why be a renter of God's goodness when you can be an owner of His amazing grace? Why stop short when you are asked to go all the way? Buy the field!

You will know you have encountered the living and loving God (and bought the field) when your ordinary life is wrecked and you have a craving for the extraordinary things that are hidden in the heart of God for you to uncover.

Emmanuel, God with us, changed everything. Jesus made His mark wherever He went, touching people with words and deeds that brought heaven crashing down to earth. He continues to move, and He wants to move and transform you too. We live in a time when people continually chase after the shiny and new and are quick to dispose of anything old. But I propose that the majesty of God is found in old things *becoming* new, not in the old being thrown away for the new.

Imagine driving down the road when suddenly you see a car with a shape, style, and sound that resemble something from a 1950s James Dean movie. It's a sleek, bubble-shaped car with a perfect hard-shelled, candy-apple-red body and a clean white racing stripe down the center. Don't you find it virtually impossible *not* to take a second look? An old car restored to mint condition commands our attention. It most definitely draws more interest than a car of the same model lying in a salvage yard somewhere, broken, busted, and discarded.

God wants to restore us. He wants to take us from the junkyard of an unrenewed life and, by His love, restore us back to our original unique, eye-catching, and commanding design. Meanwhile, He continually transforms the inner workings of our hearts, minds, and souls by the power of His amazing grace.

Long before He laid the foundations of the world, God had you in mind. Long before you had a heartbeat, He knew everything about you—the sound of your voice, your gifts and talents, and what would uniquely motivate your heart. God knew the specific time and place you would arrive to add value to the world. From the shape of your thighs to the dreams in your heart, you were intentionally molded by the hands of God. And the enemy does everything in his power to steal, kill, and destroy your beautiful design and the image of the holy God in you.

GOD'S RENOVATION PROJECT

I have personally experienced Satan's thievery, specifically when it comes to my body. After a few years of passionate involvement in the fitness industry, I was doing everything I could to be a model of health and fitness so others might invest in my passion. Yet I became sensitive to the fact that I was lacking something—breasts! Although God had blessed me with an athletic build to go with my passion and call, no matter how hard I trained, I was never going to be able to increase my breast size. As a matter of fact, since breast tissue is primarily made up of fat, the more I trained, the more that goal seemed out of reach. Every time I looked in the mirror (something we fitness trainers do a lot), the internal accusation *You look like a boy!* became louder and louder and my discontent grew stronger and stronger. During the late nineties, breast augmentation surgery was becoming more common, especially among female fitness pros who justified the surgery as no different from any other investment a professional would make in her personal growth and development.

All temptations are rooted in lies. Any temptation that goes unchecked and isn't exposed as a lie will grow into a desire. Desire, given enough time and brain space, eventually becomes an action.

With my unrenewed mind, I fell into Satan's trap, and he convinced me to hijack my original physical design.

In 1999, I went under the knife and woke up from anesthesia transformed from a double A to a C cup. It might surprise you to know that I remember instantly feeling different—not different in a "This is awesome!" kind of way but in a "This is weird" way.

I spent the next fifteen years looking more like a woman than I ever had, filling out my dresses a little more, and having the more "perfect" body, and yet . . . getting implants did not fill the ache in my soul or help the sadness and anger in my heart. Only the love of Jesus did that. And the more I fell in love with God, the more I began to realize those plastic orbs inside me weren't me. They hadn't been given by God. The deceiver had offered them to me, and I had believed his twisted tale that I was not enough without them.

In 2015, after eighteen years of growing up in my true identity as a child of God and fifteen years of carrying around what felt like two lies inside my chest, I sensed God, my good, good Father, inviting me to bravely return to my original design and come back to my whole self by removing my breast implants. He was inviting me to take back what the enemy had stolen, to be restored in my body as well as my soul. It's important that I make clear that God was not saying He would love me more for taking them out or love me any less for keeping them in. We cannot barter for God's love.

Because I feared losing part of my femininity and wondered what other people would think, it was a death-defyingly scary road to travel with God. At the same time, I found it exhilaratingly freeing. In May 2015, I said yes to that invitation, and those two deflated silicone water balloons lie somewhere in a landfill. And let me tell you, now that I am on the other side of the hardest part—my yes—I wouldn't want it any other way. In John 10:10, Jesus was not merely entertaining humanity with a pithy statement when He said He came to give us a full and abundant life—far better than the one plastic surgery or a plastic credit card can provide.

Though I had set myself up for disappointment by thinking I'd find satisfaction and meaning in a larger cup size, I now realize I was acting out of a universal need. The eternal God, who can make all things new, has planted the desire for transformation in all our hearts.

That might be one reason why the reality television genre has been such a hit. Those shows allow us to become voyeurs of people's lives behind closed doors. We enjoy watching an average-looking person become gorgeous by the power of a makeover. Several years ago, *Extreme Makeover: Home Edition* gained a massive audience by showcasing the renovation of run-down, beaten-up, mangy homes into beautiful dwelling places for families who really needed them. To me, the concept of dramatic home rehab projects is a great picture of who we are before we put our faith in Christ and who we become as we begin to open our lives to Him. Our hearts, minds, souls, and bodies have been kicked around by a fallen world, and we are like homes in need of major repairs. We all need love makeovers.

Without Christ, the homes of our inner lives—our hearts, minds, and souls—are dilapidated and in ruins. On the outside, we may look good, but inside, we're a stressed-out mess. On the days when we're anxious and afraid, our inner lives may feel more like bomb shelters than sanctuaries. On the days when we want to impress others with who we are and what we have, our inner lives may feel more like museums than cozy retreats. Meanwhile, the foundations of our homes are sinking, our wood frames are rotting, termites have infiltrated the walls, the plumbing is shot, and mold is growing behind the wallpaper. It is worse than we are willing to acknowledge; we see the evidence of ruin everywhere our spiritual eyes look.

To avoid facing our mess, we may transfer the blame onto others. Or we might focus on cleaning up just one part of ourselves—the part that everyone else can see. We are like the home owner who shoves all the junk into closets and shuts the door to every room but the living room when guests come over on short notice.

I know something of what that looks like. When I was growing up, my parents treated our house's front room like a museum for visitors. One of my mom's prized possessions was the rich avocado-green velvet couch with embellished stitching and a plastic covering (yes . . . a plastic covering) that friends noticed first when they walked into the house. Although Mom ran a tight ship and kept the house tidy, the front room was pretty much off-limits in all ways, always. I can't remember using that room as anything other than a mausoleum-like passageway for company as they journeyed to the back of our home, particularly the den, where my brother and I lay on the green shag carpet, six inches from the television, eating potato chips.

We all have a "front room" in our inner lives as well. This is the side of ourselves we manage to keep clean and presentable. It's possible we keep the outside of our houses, our bodies, looking great too. We may convince ourselves that our homes are good enough because we get to live as we wish, even though we privately long for so much more. In the quiet of our hearts, in the stillness of the night, we sense a pull toward something greater. For a time, we may convince ourselves that, given enough resources, we could make our lives so much more on our own.

But one day we realize that, like an old, neglected building that is eventually condemned, this remodel job is too big for us to do on our own. We hit a crisis or sense a yawning emptiness, and it feels as if the bank of the world has slapped yellow tape around our hearts and sent us the foreclosure notice. When we look around in desperation, we will find Jesus. He shows up and writes the check, paying our debt and redeeming our homes (our lives) so we are free and clear. But there is one string attached: Our homes no longer belong to us. They belong to God, and He has some great plans to implement in our lives.

He is not seeking to strip us of our personalities, but He is inviting us to join with Him in this grand restoration project. Jesus told His disciples, "Live in me. Make your home in me just as I do in you. In the same way that a branch can't bear grapes by itself but only by being joined to the vine, you can't bear fruit unless you are joined with me" (John 15:4, MSG).

Once the Holy Spirit takes up residence in us, He begins turning our bodies into the home, the resting place, of God. We make our home in Him, and He makes His home in us. It's mutual and reciprocal. And even if in a time of unbelief we pack our bags and leave the sanctuary He is creating, He has no plans of moving out. He won't change His mind. Christ signed the deed to our houses, our lives, in His blood. He has no plans to void that contract and leave us bankrupt and on the streets.

When you become uncomfortable with the spotlight God shines into your corners, remember that He has great plans for this place, far greater than anything you could imagine or design. After all, He created the original blueprints, and because He loves you so much, He paid a high price for you. In His grace, God wants to take you from salvation (God saving you from you) to restoration (giving you back the true you) and then move you toward transformation (turning you into the Christlike new you, built on the solid foundation of the real and restored you).

Jesus doesn't always get right to work on us with a wrecking ball—although sometimes He finds it necessary. He is patient and begins to spend time with us so He can hear our desires too. He wants to build a reconstructed relationship on vision, love, and an ultimate trust that God will give us nothing short of His best, which is far better than our idea of what's best. He created us with our own unique gifts and talents, and He doesn't want to change or remove those; that would be crazy! It would destroy His original design and work of art. He does, however, desire to strengthen those foundational traits and restore them to their natural luster and shine. Initially, all this sounds great. We are so grateful to have been saved from condemnation that we are willing partners in God's work. For the first time, we have real rest in our homes. We begin to trust that someone else sees value in this old house and will help us restore it.

Then what happens? In a hard moment or circumstance, unbelief rears its ugly head. It's as if He asked if we smelled something rotten coming from our back bedrooms and then had the nerve to offer to take a look. *Jesus is getting a little too close for comfort,* we think, *and I don't seem to be getting what I once did. He has been getting kind of pushy—and now He's just rude. How dare He! Why doesn't He just fix things and leave me alone?*

In our fear of Him uncovering any other bad smells, we may get to work around our houses. It buys us some time. Or we may throw our hands up in the air and think, *Who cares! I don't care if this house ever changes. I am totally comfortable with the way things are!*

But that odor just won't go away; in fact, it seems to be coming from several sources. Because Jesus wants to tend to that stink in our homes, He asks to see one room, then another room, and another room. Finally, He asks to see all the rooms in our homes. He is going to see the evidence of what once went on in those rooms. He is going to ask some questions, not because He doesn't know the answers but because He wants us to know, and truthfully, we are scared.

It's not just the shame of feeling "found out" if we allow God full access to the homes of our hearts; we fear we may lose the right to go back into those dark rooms to do as we wish. We may be aware that there is nothing in our hearts that God doesn't already know, but we struggle with our desire to control the process. We may give Him free access to one room but then quickly run to close off another room. His work is delayed by our diversionary tactics. We are in a salvation slump, circling the drain of our stinking thinking while trying to keep God in a box. Yet He is patient. He waits and waits, watching us busy ourselves with fluffing the pillows and tidying up around the junk and the stink in our homes, while the stench of death fills the air.

Heart disease, whether it be physical or spiritual, is killing the body of Christ. Many nominal Christians run around closing the doors in the homes of their hearts. Anger, bitterness, disappointment, and unbelief sabotage the abundant life God wants to give us. We kind of stink and we know it. And God smells it too. God sees the hurt we drag around every day, all because we refuse to stop fighting the wrong battles and join Him in the one we were made for: the battle for freedom in us and faith on the earth.

If you are struggling with your weight or obsessing over your body, most likely you have been closing doors because you get to do what you like behind closed doors. Pride, which prevents you from looking at the ruins and smelling the stink, is thwarting your transformation. This part of your sinful nature keeps you from depending on God.

A prideful person says, "I have it all under control. I have the answers. If I don't have the answers, I will figure out the answers. I will pay someone to get me the answers. I can fix this." In pride the "I, I, I" and the "me, me, me" is all we "see, see, see."

The frightening reality is that some will never even take the first step toward Christ because of their pride. Sure, their homes may look perfect and they may be living large, but because of their pride, they will never see the Lord's glory or enter into salvation. Others may be saved and invite Jesus into their homes, but they will continue to stumble around in their salvation slump.

Ultimately, we have three choices whenever God seeks to save or restore us: We can ask God to leave, we can continue stalling, or we can open the doors to our secret rooms. God will not force His way in, but He longs to lead us to a better way. In Isaiah 43:18-19, God tells the Israelites, "Forget the former things; do not dwell on the past. See, I am doing a new thing! Now it springs up; do you not perceive it? I am making a way in the wilderness and streams in the wasteland." He wants to do the same for us. Will we continue living in the wasteland, or will we make way for His streams to flow through the dry and arid places of our hearts?

Every day and through every circumstance, God is hammering in new framing, getting rid of the termites, reinstalling drywall to get rid of the mold, adding adequate lighting where there was once darkness, and applying fresh, clean-smelling paint. Before we know it, He will restore our homes to what He always intended them to be.

Once we are restored, we feel comfortable, and our anxiety dissipates. From an engineering perspective, the blueprints have been fulfilled, the house looks solid and complete, and God is pleased with the progress. At this point, it is tempting to call the work finished. We tell Jesus, "It's good enough. Look how far we have come. Let's just slow down and enjoy the fruits of our labor." Our fears, our need for comfort and control, and our selfishness prevent God from moving ahead with His transformational work and conforming us to Christ.

When it comes to our health, of course, we all desire transformation. A driving force behind our desire to move more and eat less is the hope that "in just a few short weeks you, too, can have the body you've always dreamed of!" We have all heard that promise, and if we have disconnected God from our health, we fall for it hook, line, and sinker. In our halfhearted living, we would rather paint the house and plant some flowers out front than rebuild the house from the ground up.

God has better plans for us than just giving us comfort. He wants us to have *shalom*, which is a Hebrew word that means "completeness, soundness, welfare, peace."[17] Although God is happy to see us living in a place of safety and comfort, He wants to give us more. The apostle Paul notes that "he who began a good work in you will carry it on to completion until the day of Christ Jesus" (Philippians 1:6). He knows the plans He has for us, which include "hope and a future" (Jeremiah 29:11). He wants to do for us abundantly and immeasurably more than we could ask or imagine (see Ephesians 3:20).

But even as you seek to improve your health and well-being, you must give priority to your inner life, the place where you and God meet. You will reap lasting change when you allow God full access to all the rooms of your heart's home. Why should you deny access to the One who has known you since before He formed you in the womb (see Jeremiah 1:5)? He wants to finish what He started.

Our transformation is possible only because of Jesus, which explains why the Greek word for *transform* occurs only in the New Testament. He alone can give us the ability to experience and reflect the fullness of God in our earthly lives. We are given the right to be transformed to resemble

**EVEN AS YOU SEEK TO IMPROVE YOUR HEALTH AND WELL-BEING,
YOU MUST GIVE PRIORITY TO YOUR INNER LIFE,
THE PLACE WHERE YOU AND GOD MEET.**

Jesus—God incarnate—God in the flesh. We have the right to look in the mirror and see someone who is perfect in Christ and being made perfect in a messy world, holy and whole.

When we open ourselves to God's work in our lives, not only does He restore our true identities—as His children designed to walk with Him in the cool of the day (see Genesis 3:8)—He gives us authority over all creation until His goodness, reign, and rule reach all corners of the earth.

In other words, as we are restored, Jesus invites us to look outward. Just before His crucifixion, He left this final instruction with His disciples: "Love each other as I have loved you" (John 15:12). He wants us to become His hands and feet. He wants our love to overflow from the intimate relationship between Him and us so that others may be able to walk in "newness of life" too (Romans 6:4, ESV). As we live out the greatest commandment to love God with all our hearts, souls, minds, and strength, we are changed from the inside out. When we live as personally and uniquely favored ones who are loved by God and have access to the resources of heaven, we are changed. We live as sons and daughters rather than as slaves, freely giving away what we have. As we obey the second commandment to love others, the beautiful process of salvation, restoration, and transformation can begin again in those around us.

Transformation takes God's salvation plan for the world to its final destination. God wants to see faith increase on the earth, and He plans to use people to make it happen. Willing people. People who are no longer satisfied to splash around in the shallow end of the salvation pool, content knowing that God has saved them from sin. Rather than spending time wishing for smaller thighs and flatter stomachs, these people care about the people drowning in the kiddie pool. They tell others that God wants to redeem and restore them too.

Your testimony may give others a vision for how God can also make their lives new. His hope is that others might see you and ask, "What happened to you?" and that your reply might be "I met Jesus and gave Him my heart and my body too!"

Because the goal of transformation is to make us like Christ, we must remember that our internal remodeling project won't be complete until we leave this earth. When we see God starting over in an area we thought we had finished fixing up, we must exhale and trust Him. God is not like a difficult, scheming contractor. He's actually fun to work with. Join in and whistle while He works. When you trust Him to remake every room, He will turn your heart into a masterpiece of His glory.

Whenever you open your heart to God, He works in you to bring about the changes you cannot make on your own to get you to your promised land. The transformation journey is an adventure. Keep your adventuresome spirit alive! Travel with God from one season of life into another. Some seasons will be intense, filled with resistance. Engage your core (both the center of your physical self and the values you hold), keep your eyes on Christ, and lean into the struggle. The storm will not last forever, and you will find yourself on the other side of that tempest in a more spacious land. Keep moving to keep growing. Keep growing into that royal robe of righteousness in which God draped you when you first professed Jesus as your King. You live a life of nobility, and favor follows you wherever you go.

Some days you may feel as if all you are doing is sitting on the ground banging nails into a two-by-four while He operates the heavy machinery. Remember that He lovingly looks at you and cheers, "Good job, My child! I love what you are doing! Keep going. You're getting it!"

RESPOND

With All Your Heart

> You're doing a great job working your way through the Wellness Revelation
> Workout Calendar (see page 240). Keep going! You're changing on the inside
> now. When you feel like you don't have the energy, ask God for the grace to
> help you in your time of weakness.

If anyone is in Christ, the new creation has come:
The old has gone, the new is here!

2 CORINTHIANS 5:17

Since you've made it to week 7, I can say with confidence that you are not the same person who began this journey. If you can't see it right now, it's probably because you forgot to put on your gospel goggles this morning. Go ahead and put them on so you can prepare your heart and mind to respond to the following training assignment.

Take a moment to be still and breathe. Ask the Holy Spirit to guide you into all truth. Then, on the left side of the next page, write down all the things the old you believed about living a healthy and whole life. On the right side of the page, write down everything the new you believes about what it means to live healthy, whole, and *free*!

Old

Example: *I'm so tired tonight that I think I'll skip working out and just watch the TV pilot I read about on Facebook.*

New

Example: *I know I won't want to head to the gym after work tomorrow if I go home first, so I'll pack my gear tonight and take it with me in the morning.*

RENEW

With All Your Soul

We cannot forget that God's desire has always been for an intimate and loving relationship with us. His plan has always been to win us back by the greatness of His love. Wherever He dwells, His presence and holiness reside. He says, "I am the LORD, who brought you up out of Egypt to be your God; therefore be holy, because I am holy" (Leviticus 11:45).

Why did God rescue the Israelites from bondage and slavery? Because He loved them. Why did He want them to be holy? Because wherever God takes up residence, things must be right, true, and glorious, for He is worthy. In this week's Bible study, let's look at what Scripture has to say about transformation and about becoming new creations in Christ, so that *His* holiness and glory may reign and *our* joy may be made complete.

1. In God's quest to restore us to right relationship with Him, He offers us a three-step makeover. It begins with salvation (saving you from you), is followed by restoration (giving you back the true you), and finally moves into transformation (making you more Christlike). Would you say He is nudging you toward one of these steps, or are you and God actively participating together in one of these stages? Explain.

2. Read Ephesians 5:1-2. How does the apostle Paul describe how God the Father perceived Christ's sacrifice on our behalf? How does that change the way we "smell"?

3. Please read 2 Corinthians 2:14-17. With a humble heart, remember the "stink" inside us that we discussed in this week's reading. Take some time to meditate and reflect on anything putrid in your own heart. What stink in your life do you think God wants to remove?

4. Verses 15 and 16 tell us that we are the aroma of God. Who likes the way we smell and who does not? Why?

5. In verse 14, Paul talks about Christ's "triumphal procession." He is drawing on imagery from a Roman ceremony called the Triumph, in which a victorious general was honored with a festive, ceremonial parade through the streets of Rome. The parade would feature incense-burning censers, and flower petals would be strewn and then crushed under the horses' feet, giving off a powerful aroma that filled the city. John MacArthur said, "By analogy, every believer is *transformed* and called by the Lord to be an influence for His gospel throughout the world" (emphasis mine).[18] Name one way in which you can be a sweet-smelling fragrance that draws people to Christ this week.

6. Read 2 Corinthians 3:1-6. In verses 1 through 3, Paul compares believers not to a fragrance but to a letter that testifies to Christ's work in their lives. If your life were a letter testifying to the Spirit's work in your life, what would it say?

7. Weight-loss and other health and fitness trends can lead to very selfish attitudes. We are quick to become self-confident once we start seeing results or have reached our goals. This is why it is essential for us to stay confident in only *one* thing: the power of God to change what needs to be changed in our lives—*His* power in *our* dwelling space.

   Read verses 4-6. Note that Paul places no confidence in himself; his confidence comes only from God. Describe a time when you put too much confidence in yourself.

8. Read 2 Corinthians 3:11-16. What is the purpose of the veil mentioned in verse 13? Why did God have Moses wear it whenever Moses had been in His presence?

9. According to verses 14 and 15, who wears the veil today? What two parts of their bodies is it covering? According to verse 16, what happens when someone turns to the Lord?

10. Read 2 Corinthians 3:17-18. Once the veil is lifted, we are empowered by the Spirit. According to these verses, what always accompanies Him? How does Paul describe the Spirit's work in our lives?

Dear Jesus,

I want You to change me, but first I must let go of the fear that tells me it is too scary, that I cannot trust You, that I will fail, and that I know better than You. Please help me to trust You, to trust Your plans for my life, and to trust that You want to make me holy and whole. I desire transformation and for the stink in my heart to be removed. Speak to me each day, letting me know when I am getting in the way of Your love makeover for my life.
✝ Amen.

RELATE

With All Your Mind and Strength

The following questions are designed to help you apply all you've learned this week to your fitness journey. Get with your accountability partner or small group and work honestly through these questions. Consider journaling your answers with God before sharing with your partner or group.

1. What stinking thinking tends to push you into a salvation slump? What is God teaching you to help you move past these holding patterns in your life?

2. What areas of your life and personal character is God renovating? How would you describe the ways He's restoring His original design for you?

3. How is God transforming you into greater Christlikeness?

4. Picture your life as a house where God dwells. What kinds of things would people notice if they walked into your home today? What is the vision for your home in the future?

5. How do you see food and exercise fitting into God's plan for your personal transformation? What is He teaching you about them?

RECIPROCATE

A Divine Appointment

by Breanne Morrow,
Revelation Wellness Ambassador

When I was nineteen, I began working as a dancer in a strip club. For five years, my life was filled with reckless sex, drug use, and partying. After leaving an abusive relationship, I met the man of my dreams, who was a devoted Christian. I walked away from the dancer life because I wanted a real chance with this "good guy." We've since married and have two young children.

I recommitted my life to Christ and was baptized in 2012. That same year, my church introduced me to the Divine ministry, an outreach to women in the sex industry, and I became a volunteer. Every other month we visit the fourteen strip clubs in Orange County, California, where we distribute gifts for the dancers, as well as the phone number for our hotline.

As I reached out to women in the two strip clubs where I once worked, God began to open my eyes to the lies I believed. I thought that I'd been created to be used by men and that love came from their acceptance. I also believed that by using my body, I could stay in control and get love when I needed it. I thought I was different from the other dancers because I wasn't as visibly "messed up" as they were. Through the Divine ministry, God showed me I was just like them in my brokenness. I needed to allow Jesus to penetrate my heart even more so I could truly love these women.

I now understand that true love comes from the Lord. I cannot love others without first receiving His love myself. The women I meet through Divine will continue in their lifestyle until they know their value and worth as God's precious daughters as well.

In June 2014, we received a late-night call from Nicole, a woman who had gotten our number the previous week in one of our gift bags. She had only begun dancing about two months before. She had taken pole dancing fitness classes and thought it'd be fun to do and a good way to make some extra money.

Nicole was also the single mom of a little girl, and she felt alone and wanted to talk with someone. We spoke for about forty-five minutes. Then I offered to pray with her, and she accepted. I told her she could call or text me anytime.

A few weeks later Nicole called again. She was worried because a customer had offered her two thousand dollars if she would meet him outside the club for coffee. She thought perhaps he planned to kidnap her and asked what I thought she should do. I recommended she stop all contact with him immediately.

She began to cry and said she didn't want to dance anymore. In fact, since that conversation, Nicole never went back to dancing. Instead, she rededicated her life to Christ, was baptized (by me!), and continues to grow in the Word and her relationship with our Lord and Savior. I am so grateful for the opportunity to tell women like Nicole about the redeeming love of Christ.

PRESS ON

Not that I have already obtained all this, or have already arrived at my goal,
but I press on to take hold of that for which Christ Jesus took hold of me.

PHILIPPIANS 3:12

For the past seven weeks, you have dedicated yourself to a new way of life— a healthy and whole way. And it hasn't been easy. That is because anything worth having in life always comes at a price. People who pay nothing, value nothing. You have paid the price. You have overcome temptation. No doubt you have woken up with sore muscles and still directed yourself to move, sweat, and eat right for another day. You have gone to bed with a tummy that is half-full instead of stuffed. You are learning the art of sufficiency.

Or perhaps you don't feel as if you've paid any price in the pursuit of wellness and wholeness. If that is your situation, I invite you to allow the Spirit to search you and reveal where things got off track. Don't fall into the trap of taking on any shame. Simply consider whether you are willing to turn back to page 1 and begin again. Whenever you find yourself returning to your old comfortable ways, take a moment to catch your breath and get back in step with the Spirit. You didn't miss God's call, and He didn't ditch you. He is eager to walk with you and show you the way. Remember that you are truly, madly, and deeply loved by a God who will go to any lengths to see you seated at His banquet table. Your worth has been settled. The Cross says you are worth it all!

Perhaps you have been pleasantly surprised at the way you've already been able to incorporate healthy eating and workout habits into your daily life. As much as I would love to pat you on the back and say, "Well done. You did it!" I would be setting you up with a false sense of security.

If you are achieving success, don't allow yourself to wander. Keep your mind and heart focused on God. As soon as you or I think we have "arrived" and have it under control, pride develops, which leads to rebellion. Lasting health and wholeness, which lie in holiness, require interdependence with God, not independence from Him.

In eight weeks of pursuing a healthy and whole life, a gospel-centered life, you are just beginning to plant the seeds and tend to your field. Perhaps you see fresh green buds of hope sprouting forth and are tempted to get comfortable. Now is not the time to let up. A harvest is coming! And until we step into our glorified selves and see Jesus face-to-face, we can never fully relax. Rest assured there will be seasons of rest, but this is not to be confused with seasons of gluttony or self-centered living. Day by day, glory to glory, faith to faith, we must continue to sow the good seeds of physical, emotional, mental, and spiritual health.

I refuse to set you up for disappointment by telling you that training for and sustaining a lifestyle of wellness will get easier. However, while it won't necessarily be effortless, it will become more familiar. Your new normal can become a daily life lived inside the supernatural home of God's Kingdom. It takes time for us to learn the new house rules there—to trust that healthy living is part of the love, power, and freedom our Father wants us to have. It takes time for former orphans to understand what it means to live in our Father's house, where we have access to a refrigerator full of good eats and we have a bedroom that will never be turned into an office. It takes time to mature into sons and daughters of the King rather than slaves to our own desires.

Twenty-plus years ago when I first opened my heart to King Jesus, I expected that in no time flat I would be living in the land of milk and honey and all would be right with the world. Jesus had rescued me, all right, but it wasn't to make me comfortable. Yes, He redeemed me so that I might have the same Kingdom privileges and access to His Father that He possesses. But He also saved me to send me out to battle—a battle that I most assuredly will win because He settled the outcome at Calvary.

I have been extravagantly blessed and endlessly challenged as I've followed Christ. When I recently prayed, asking God why following Him seems so hard, I sensed Him reminding me, *Alisa, you are getting My Way confused with My*

Remember to use your Moving Forward Journal this week to track your food and water intake, as well as to remain focused on this week's Scripture verse. You can download a copy at www.revelationwellness.org/book/workout or photocopy the template on page 239.

Work. Then He brought to mind Matthew 11:30, where Jesus says that His yoke, or my work, is easy and light, and Matthew 7:13-14, where He says that His Way is narrow and small and few will find it. In other words, the path God leads me on will be treacherous because the enemy will do everything he can to block the Way from people who haven't yet found it. The enemy wants to get in the way of the Way to try to convince me that God is not good. However, when I abide in Jesus, I can count on Him to make His work in me light. In that quiet moment with God, I felt Him say, *Stay easy and light, Alisa. Abide in Me and I will abide in you. Together, you and I will work to clear the Way so others can find it and follow Me too. But remember, I get to do all the heavy lifting. The Way will be hard, but the work is easy and light.*

As you continue making healthy lifestyle choices, don't forget that the enemy, the world, and your flesh will tempt you either to indulge yourself or to fixate on healthy food and exercise. Remember the two clients I introduced you to in the beginning of this book? The one begins strong, only to lose her focus and become obsessed with her body. The other begins strong, only to lose focus and give up.

If we are not intentional about walking with God in our pursuit of wellness, we will almost certainly fall into one of these two traps. If we begin making healthy lifestyle changes but then begin depending on food and leisure for our peace rather than on God, we will be enticed again by our old idol and comforter, food. If we merely exchange the idol of too much food and not enough exercise for too little food and too much exercise, we will shove God out of the picture and never get a chance to enter the rest He wants to give us. Either way, we will miss out on His holy contentment and His promise to "meet all [our] needs according to the riches of his glory in Christ Jesus" (Philippians 4:19).

You'll encounter fewer barriers in your quest for health and wholeness if you follow the counsel of the apostle Paul: "Continue to work out your salvation with fear and trembling, for it is God who works in you to will and to act in order to fulfill his good purpose" (Philippians 2:12-13). At first glance, this Scripture makes us think that we had better keep working hard and keep things moving in the right direction or God will be unhappy with us. But Paul quickly reminds us that although we are to continue obeying and following Him, we don't do the work. God does! He is for you! He wants to see the impact of your goodness grow! He wants you to take back anything your family of origin forfeited.

So what, then, is our work? It is to continue to let God do the work in us. We give God 24-7 permission to search us, know us, and teach us about His goodness. When the enemy tries to use insurmountable obstacles or painful circumstances to keep us from the joy of our salvation, we are to keep seeking God. In those hard times, our work is to let God's love work its way into us so our fear and unbelief will work their way out of us.

Seek the Spirit throughout your day. And when you hear His voice, do what He asks! His work in you is easy and light even when the Way feels hard. We are a "living sacrifice" (Romans 12:1), people who breathe, think, feel, speak, and act in accordance with love. We must persevere in the Way and let God do His work.

YOUR ATTITUDE TO CARRY ON

The attitude of disciples who are growing in holy, whole, and wholehearted living is rooted in humility. Humble people do not live in timidity and fear, thinking and living small because they are afraid that they might steal God's glory. God is not afraid of us stealing anything from Him. God's not afraid, period. So neither should we be, as image bearers of a holy God. Humble hearts belong to people who have been so wrecked by God's love that they are willing to allow Him to extinguish all the selfish, burning desires of their hearts so they can live according to the Spirit. They know that their flesh apart from God's presence is grossly destructive but that their body partnered with God's presence is wonderfully powerful!

Humble-hearted people fear one thing: the absence of God. This is why David, a man after God's own heart, a mighty and humble warrior, cried out for two things: (1) that he could be in God's presence and (2) that God would never take away His presence:

> One thing I ask from the LORD, this only do I seek: that I may dwell in the house of the LORD all the days of my life, to gaze on the beauty of the LORD and to seek him in his temple.
>
> PSALM 27:4

> Do not cast me from your presence or take your Holy Spirit from me. Restore to me the joy of your salvation and grant me a willing spirit, to sustain me.
>
> PSALM 51:11-12

When you have an attitude of humility, you are willing to learn and grow as God works within you, even when He is challenging you to overcome your spirit of fear and timidity. God will ensure that you come face-to-face with what frightens you most. It's His way of showing you that fear has always been an illusion projected onto the walls of your unbelieving heart. Do not be afraid! His saving love will deliver you, moving you from where you are now to where He wants you to go. His ways will not be comfortable, but they will be best.

In reality, what choice do we have but to follow Him? We know where we have been and how unsatisfying those places are. We can choose to turn back and return to our old, comfortable ways, or we can continue down this humble, narrow, hard road, knowing that God will use it for His good purposes on the earth, as well as for our good and the good of others.

Humility is hard in part because it asks us to think of others as more important than ourselves.

Do nothing out of selfish ambition or vain conceit. Rather, in humility value others above yourselves, not looking to your own interests but each of you to the interests of the others.

PHILIPPIANS 2:3-4

Say what? That's so unnatural. It doesn't feel right—kind of like the experience of getting older. Lately I've noticed my body changing. Gravity is having its way. Time marches on, and its muddy army boots seem to be treading right over my body and leaving marks. Some days I see crevices, crags, and sags in my face when I look in the mirror. *You're old*, I tell myself. *You're losing it.* (Whatever "it" is.) *You're not as* [fill in the blank] *as you once were.* So I push, pull, stretch, and squeeze my face, hoping to spot my younger self. I would be lying if I told you I never wrestle with the temptation to take a shortcut. Some days I can almost convince myself that a few needle injections of neurotoxins and short-term facial paralysis don't seem outside of the freedom we have in Christ. And maybe they're not. But something stops me . . . the thought of others.

The thought of my daughter stops me. What kind of message would I be sending her about aging if I tried to reverse it in myself? What messages of inadequacy might I be sending to aging women who can't afford regular trips to a plastic surgeon? The thought of you, reading this book, stops me. I am passionate about seeing you find *real* freedom to live true to your authentic self in Christ, not based on what is seen but on what is unseen (see 2 Corinthians 4:16-18). The pursuit of perfection is an easy prison to enter but a hard one to leave.

The truth is, the aging process happens to everyone, everywhere. However, modern Western culture has voted and the results are in . . . getting old is unacceptable! Growing older, which some cultures hold in high esteem, has been pooh-poohed and made taboo in our society. We value preserving the body and pursuing perfection over persevering in the good, kind, noble, and true. I am craving what is real and true! How about you?

When I take a moment in humility to bow my heart before the presence of the Lord, I realize that getting older, especially growing in the Lord, is an honor and a privilege. I remember how I earned each of the lines on my face and how they help me tell the story of God's faithfulness to me. I have cried. I have laughed. I have furrowed my brow in distress. Every time, God came through. So in the moments when I look at those lines and think, *I can fix this*, God enables me to sober up to the real battle for which I was born—the battle for freedom. I want to see my daughter embrace this freedom, along with other daughters of the King who yearn to know they have been chosen and are always enough. I also want real men to rise, hunger, and fight for the freedom of real women who cannot be bought, bartered, or conformed into artificial beings. I find more life by giving up on my shortcuts to life. Yes, it is good practice to consider others before ourselves. Doing so keeps us humble, courageous, and kind.

Be careful when you are tempted to return to your old way of thinking—whether you tend toward self-criticism or pride. Recognize the temptation and don't move until you can catch your breath. Groan, breathe, and stay in God's presence, where the truth of His Word keeps you free.

Advertisements, social media, and sometimes even our friends lure us to look to this or that for help rather than to God. Before we know it, we have hired a personal trainer, severely restricted our calories, or spent multiple hours at the gym, all in the name of willpower and self-control. This is nothing new. As God was preparing His people to enter the Promised Land, He warned them: "Be careful, or you will be enticed to turn away and worship other gods and bow down to them. Then the Lord's anger will burn against you, and he will shut up the heavens so that it will not rain and the ground will yield no produce, and you will soon perish from the good land the Lord is giving you" (Deuteronomy 11:16-17).

Sometimes trouble comes not because you look to others to save you, but because you look to yourself. When you place your heart and desires higher

WHENEVER YOU FIND YOURSELF RETURNING TO YOUR OLD COMFORTABLE WAYS, TAKE A MOMENT TO CATCH YOUR BREATH AND GET BACK IN STEP WITH THE SPIRIT.

than the heart of God, you have become proud. When you find yourself in your own crazy because you are looking to other people or yourself for direction, don't fall into hopelessness! Celebrate that you recognize that you are in a bad place.

If you are not intentional about walking with God, you will run ahead of Him. When I realize I've lost my humility, I recognize it as my cue to go to my secret place with the Lord. It may even be a mobile secret place. Often I sit in my car, put on music, and sing. Or I simply sit in silence. I *remember* what God has said to me. I open His Word and reinforce His words to me by reciting His promises back to Him. I let God catch up to me and wrap me in His affection. My primary goal is to receive His love, and His love sets me straight. Sometimes this process of getting my humility back only takes a few minutes, and sometimes it takes a few days. But I have no intention of changing my heart's affections. I will not give my heart to any other god. My God is good, faithful, and kind, and He will come through and deliver me.

HAVE A GOD-CENTERED PLAN

As important as humility is, you will also need a plan as you move ahead. This reflects God, who created us in His image: "God is not a God of confusion but of peace" (1 Corinthians 14:33, ESV). We, too, are well served when we have a plan—a God-centered plan—and with humility, we hold it loosely. The key is allowing Him to lead the way.

When God laid it on my heart to partner with Him in the field of fitness and wellness, all I sensed Him telling me was "Weigh less to feed more" (the original title of this book). That was all the direction I got. But that started a fire in me that could not be put out. Though I had no idea what this program was supposed to look like, I knew that God was asking me to *do something*! And so I did. I got right to work making big plans and setting lofty goals. But as I tossed over and over in my mind how this ministry might take shape, I began losing my peace. No matter how hard I worked or how much I planned, I felt no peace.

Then one day it hit me: I was doing this all on my own terms with my own ideas and goals. I had run ahead of God. No wonder I felt exhausted! I realized that my plans can't support the goodness His plans can. I was so busy showing God what I could do that I never asked Him what He wanted to do and when He wanted to do it. I had left God in the dust.

I exhaled and found my peace. I asked Him for His will to be done, and I waited for Him to speak before I moved. In time, God gave me another piece of the vision. Soon momentum began to build. To this day, I have to remind myself to take my hands off my life. If God decides to move in another direction, I will be ready to follow. Do you see why a humble heart is necessary? Waiting may seem unproductive, yet the apostle Paul explains why it is so critical:

Everyone who competes in the games goes into strict training. They do it to get a crown that will not last, but we do it to get a crown that will last forever. Therefore I do not run like someone running aimlessly; I do not fight like a boxer beating the air. No, I strike a blow to my body and make it my slave so that after I have preached to others, I myself will not be disqualified for the prize.

I CORINTHIANS 9:25-27

God is less concerned about change in our outer lives than He is about change in our inner lives. The more our desires change to align with God's will, the more we will be living for an eternal crown filled with jewels like love, peace, trust, obedience, purity, and grace.

Paul did not "run like someone running aimlessly" or "fight like a boxer beating the air." He had a plan! He focused on God and went into strict training so that nothing would sidetrack him. He fought for his right to be holy and whole so that nothing would disqualify him from hearing, "Well done, good and faithful servant! You have been faithful with a few things; I will put you in charge of many things. Come and share your master's happiness!" (Matthew 25:23).

Just like Paul, I charge you to think of yourself as an athlete, with clear eyes and open ears. Go into strict training for the purposes of God. A God-centered plan keeps the will of God as the goal. A plan to develop bigger biceps or thinner thighs isn't terrible in and of itself, but without the purposes of God at the center, that goal could turn us into carrot-chasing rabbits who run in nauseating circles. It's wise for us to check our hearts with God when making any plans or goals to be sure they are from Him and are not our attempt to force Him to give us what we want, when we want it. Just as I initially ran ahead of God when I sensed Him calling me to write this book, any plans we make that move ahead of God or any work we do without the approval of God will lack His provision. Don't waste your time or add any hurt to your life—seek God's plan and wait on His timing.

PARTY LIKE JESUS!

Christ loved the church and gave himself up for her . . . having cleansed her by the washing of water with the word, so that he might present the church to himself in splendor, without spot or wrinkle or any such thing, that she might be holy and without blemish.

EPHESIANS 5:25-27, ESV

Diverse individuals who've come together in holy unity make up the church. And Jesus calls the church His bride. God is in love with the church, no matter what others might say. You and I are God's beloved! Uniquely and corporately, we are loved. And God is planning a big celebration party for His bride.

The apostle John offers a glimpse of that glorious feast:

"Let us rejoice and exult
    and give him the glory,
for the marriage of the Lamb has come,
    and his Bride has made herself ready;
it was granted her to clothe herself
    with fine linen, bright and pure"—

for the fine linen is the righteous deeds of the saints.

And the angel said to me, "Write this: Blessed are those who are invited to the marriage supper of the Lamb."

REVELATION 19:7-9, ESV

With that ultimate banquet in mind, I want to close by giving you one more picture of the proper place of food in the abundant life that comes from knowing God's love and His heart of celebration. Please ignite your imagination with me for a moment.

You wake up one gorgeous Saturday morning. The sky is cobalt blue, sprinkled with stark white puffy clouds. You spring out of bed filled with great anticipation.

You begin your usual morning routine: a healthy breakfast of eggs on toast with a warm cup of coffee. With your Bible and breakfast in hand, you head out to your favorite spot on the deck. *What a great day!* you keep thinking. Once the eggs have settled in your stomach and God's Word has filled your heart, you lace up your running shoes and head out for a walk or jog. Breathing the fresh air in and out, you sense the Lord's pleasure on your life. Joy is fueling your movement. It feels as if the wind is at your back no matter what direction you run.

The rest of the day unfolds kindly but with growing excitement. At about four o'clock, you kick into high gear as the anticipation builds. It's time for a shower, followed by the fun of "dress up." You carefully do your hair and makeup. Your long white dress hangs in the corner with your shoes beneath it, next to a table holding jewelry fit for a queen. It's time to put the whole look together. You pull on one layer at a time, and slowly the reflection in the mirror transfigures into the image of a woman who is most beautiful. A woman who is royalty.

By 5:30 p.m. you are ready. A long, shiny black car pulls up and whisks you off to the church. You head to a private room where friends and loved ones wait for you. Your beauty takes everyone's breath away, and you see tears of joy in the eyes of people you love. Tangible excitement fills the room.

Then the big moment comes when you walk to the doors of the sanctuary. The organist pulls out all the stops and hits that robust C chord, the kind that commands attention. The ancient hand-carved doors swing open to reveal you—the most beautiful sight for all eyes to see.

You walk slowly but confidently to the end of the aisle, where you meet your groom, the one who will say, "I choose you. Forever and always." Together you and your beloved commit your lives to each other.

Once the ceremony is over, you and your groom are ready to celebrate! The band plays, and servers bring out trays of five-star food. The waiter comes to serve you and your groom first. Dinner looks good, and it smells even better. With all the excitement quelling your appetite, you haven't had much to eat since breakfast. You're hungry. The waiter dips over your shoulder to hand you your plate, but you say, "Nope, none for me; I am on a diet."

What?! Of course you wouldn't say that. Of course you are going to eat, drink, and be merry on a beautiful day like today. This is a celebration of goodness, for goodness' sake! And food—good food—is a part of this celebratory moment.

God gives us good food as a reflection of His heart of goodness and His Kingdom. Of course, good food is not the high point of this unforgettable day. The high point is the celebration of you and your groom coming together as one. The food plays a supporting role to the pleasure and enjoyment of love finding and having its way.

Our God is a good God, and He is into good things because He created "good." A wedding is a good thing. A birthday is a good thing. An anniversary is a good thing. The day we celebrate Jesus' birth, Christmas Day, is a good thing. Food is there to enhance the experience, but hear me when I say that food does not a celebration make. People make a celebration. Joyful hearts make a celebration. People moving together toward a common goal make all of heaven celebrate!

Because of the abundance available in the Western world, we have turned every day into a celebration of sorts. We have many reasons to celebrate, but food is never to be the focus. It can be a part of it, an enjoyable part, but it can never be the focus.

Perhaps you're thinking, *Well, Jesus was always eating with His disciples and feeding the multitudes, so we should too.* I agree. It is good for us to break bread with one another, and it is an honor to partner with God and feed the hungry. But we cannot forget that food will never permanently satisfy anyone. Everyone will be hungry again. Only Jesus can satisfy.

Jesus used food to bless others so they might come near to Him. Is food bringing you closer to God, or is it allowing you to keep a comfortable barrier between you and Him? Is Christ's love in you and on earth your main mission? Or is maintaining your waistline or filling your belly what drives you day after day?

What we all really hunger for is relationship, first with God and then with other people. We are all starving for the wedding feast—a celebration of lifelong committed love, not fast takeout from the drive-through.

This beautiful gift called life includes many celebrations and feasts. What a gift! Partake! Enjoy! But do so with a sober spirit. Keep the Spirit, the presence of God, in view, and you won't need to keep looking at the number on the scale or obey the lies that shout at your reflection in the mirror. If you wake in the morning with that "fat" feeling and an awareness that you didn't need that last piece of cake, consider yourself loved. Listen to God's voice and do not harden your heart like you did in the past. When you slip up, never put on shame or become a prisoner of hopelessness. Be ready to make a better choice the next time by calling on the power of grace. God's grace is always sufficient in the moments you are weak. Stay mindful, live wholeheartedly, and be sure to ask yourself often, *Who or what is mastering me?*

Go live this amazing free life you have been given because God so loved you! Live a life that points others toward the Way that is narrow and hard because without you helping direct others to it, very few will find it. Live so that others see that whether you eat or drink or whatever you do, you do it *all* for the glory of God.

RESPOND

With All Your Heart

> Be sure to access the Wellness Revelation Workout Calendar on page 240. Your fitness training peaks this week, so finish strong! At the end of the week, do not despise the small changes, and do not boast in the big. You are God's workmanship now: healthy, whole, and free.

GOD-CENTERED PLAN

1. As you began this journey, you created an action plan (see page 10) that included your physical and spiritual goals. Look back at those goals now. In what areas have you made progress? At this point, would you modify those goals in any way?

2. What will you do when something interferes with your goals?

3. What lasting changes in how you eat will you incorporate into your plan?

4. How many times a week do you plan to exercise? On what days and at what times? Be as specific as you can.

5. When will you set aside time each day to spend with the Lord so you can read, learn, and grow in the love found in His Word?

6. When you struggle because things feel hard, what will you do?

7. Describe your secret place where you meet with the Lord. What does it mean for you to go there?

8. To whom will you look for accountability?

MY PRAYER FOR YOU . . .

I pray that this program has planted in you a consciousness that everything you do matters: it matters to you, it matters to others, and mostly, it matters to our God. I pray that you will continue to seek God with your whole heart and to live wholeheartedly. I pray that you will love God and others and that you will allow yourself to be loved. I pray that you will continue to walk humbly with your God. I pray for a continued revelation of strength to do the seemingly impossible, finding that God is greater in you than you could ever be in yourself.

I pray you will know firsthand that His love never quits!

Alisa

RENEW

With All Your Soul

In week 6, I mentioned that Deuteronomy is a record of Moses' farewell address to the Israelites. In chapter 8, he encourages them to look back with gratitude for the many ways God had provided for them as they wandered through the desert and to look ahead with anticipation at the good gifts they would soon receive.

My hope is that in the past eight weeks you have begun to see the sprouting of a new "land" inside you—that the waters of God's grace are beginning to flow and that your soul now craves His good gifts, represented in this Scripture passage by wheat, barley, vines, fig trees, pomegranates, olive oil, and honey.

1. Read Deuteronomy 8. What does God ask us to do in our minds to prevent our hearts from getting hard? (See verse 2.)

2. Note how God used food as a means of grabbing the Israelites' hearts and captivating them. According to verse 3, what was God trying to teach the Israelites through His provision of manna?

3. Recalling God's goodness is a mental exercise that we should engage in every day. Physical exercise improves our fitness and strength; remembering who

God is renews our minds and increases our joy. In the space below, write down what God has shown you over the past eight weeks that you will choose to remember in the days and months ahead.

4. In verses 6-9, Moses goes into detail about what the "good land" God is giving the Israelites will look like, while also reminding them to observe His commands (verse 6). Moving forward, what command(s) is God asking you to observe?

5. Please write Deuteronomy 8:10 below. What does this verse reveal about the character of God? About how we should respond to Him?

6. Read verses 11-20. What will happen if we forget who God is and refuse to obey His commands? How does refusing to obey God's commands affect our health?

7. According to Deuteronomy 8:17, when we experience success, pleasure, and comfort, what are we likely to do?

8. In verse 18, Moses reminds the people that their success and wealth come from God. Could the same be said about our health? How does that perspective change the way you see your struggles with weight and health?

9. What warning appears at the end of this chapter (see verses 19-20)? How would you define an idol? What idols have you set up in your heart in the past?

10. The disciple John was known as "the disciple whom Jesus loved" (John 13:23). He spoke the language of love well. He wrote 1 John to help believers understand that "God is love" (1 John 4:16). In the very last verse (1 John 5:21), John reveals the secret of remaining centered in God's love. How would you apply his advice to your own life?

Lord Jesus,

I know that this does not end here. I am on a journey toward the heart of the Father, and I will not quit until I have taken hold of the promises You have for me in this life. Help me stay under Your umbrella of love, grace, mercy, peace, and protection. I give myself to You—all of me for You. Lord, I give You all of my heart, all of my mind, all of my soul, and all of my strength, and I ask that You make every part of me holy and whole. I confess my fear and my unbelief. Please help remove these thoughts and feelings from my heart. I am Your vessel for You to pour Yourself into. Only You will satisfy. I no longer want to hunger for anything that will not nourish me. Only You will nourish me. I am Yours. Please take me to the good land.

The disciple You love so much

RELATE

With All Your Mind and Strength

The following questions are designed to help you apply all you've learned this week to your fitness journey. Get with your accountability partner or small group and work honestly through these questions. Consider journaling your answers with God before sharing with your partner or group.

1. Last week we talked about how pride is a major stumbling block to transformation. The opposite of pride is humility. What does the word *humility* bring to mind for you? Envision a situation in the future where you will need humility to help you stay on track toward transformation and freedom in your quest for health and wholeness.

2. Do you think it is really possible to rest from your work? Have you ever felt this? Please share a time when you did.

3. If you are a follower of Jesus, He has made holiness and wholeness your birthright. However, Satan will do everything he can to take that from you. How can you guard yourself for the battle that awaits?

4. Proverbs 14:12 says, "There is a way that appears to be right, but in the end it leads to death." What, then, leads to life? If you're not sure, see Proverbs 3:5-6.

5. If you are discussing these reflection questions with a small group or accountability partner, please share your God-centered plans with one another.

6. Take some time to write your own Reciprocate story (see page 233). If you are discussing these reflection questions with a small group or accountability partner, please share your stories with one another.

RECIPROCATE

Write your own short story about a time, preferably during the last eight weeks, when lifestyle changes related to food, exercise, or Bible study gave you the energy, motivation, or opportunity to serve someone else. Be sure to include your thoughts on how God is transforming you and leading you from poverty to freedom and riches in Christ.

ACKNOWLEDGMENTS

This book was close to ten years in the making.

This book is evidence that God is real, that He really loves us, and that He calls us to do things we never thought we could. This book would not exist if it wasn't for the Voice of Love who called me out of darkness and into His marvelous light—and then asked me to bring a laptop and start writing. I was the girl who finagled her way through high school English and chose to write book reports only on books with Cliffs Notes versions, so you can imagine my anxious disbelief when God spoke and I began writing this message almost ten years ago.

This book is for God's glory alone. He called me. I wrote. Like Moses, I tried to talk Him out of it, but He would have none of that. Thank You, God, for seeing in me what I could not see. Thank You for wooing me into doing scary things. More than anything else, thank You for coming for me. Thank You for grabbing me firmly by the hand and gently leading me into an open and spacious land. I love You, for always and forever.

To my husband, Simon: In our first year of marriage, you told me, "You should write a book." I laughed. But God knew. God made you for me, and you make it possible for me to freely be me and to boldly do what God has called me to do. You stood by me in the darkest of seasons, when it seemed like a new day would never come. You're my warrior-man, my sheepdog, my confidant, and the one I want to grow old and wrinkled with. Thank you for the freedom you give me to proclaim freedom to the captives. I love you.

Jack and Sophia: You've been beyond gracious with me, your messy mama. You train me up in the ways of love. You didn't ask to be the kids of a woman who would proclaim the Good News, only to watch her up close as she struggles on bad days. But God knew you were the tough and tender ones for me. Thank you for extending to me your never-ending mercy, grace, and forgiveness. I love you, my Jacky Boy and Sophia Mia. I pray that I have paid the price and continue to pay the price for you, your children, and your children's children to be free—for a thousand generations. You are a new generation. You are free!

The Revelation Wellness core team: A special thank-you to Leah (COO extraordinaire), Heather, Carole, Chris, Fran, Kristen, Nicole, Myra, Tammy, Sara, Kara, Katrina, Courtney, Dana, Staci, Claire, Anna, Renee, Laura, and Lauren. Thank you for the sacrifices of time and energy you have made over the past months to give me the space to embark on this publishing adventure. Thank you for being a team that isn't only willing to work for a ministry about living wholly in God's love, but that also lets God do the work of wholeness in them. You are all the definition of courage and integrity. A special thank-you to Don and Renee Worcester, who sow countless seeds of loving-kindness into my family at home as well as into this team—my family on mission.

The Revelation Wellness family of instructors: We did it! You did it! You prayed this book into the hands of many, and the day has come. I know I am standing on the shoulders of your prayers, and for that, I cannot thank you enough. Thank you for continually putting yourselves and your fears on the line for the sake of our King. The way you ring your fitness freedom bell and deliver "the pizza" to hungry hearts helps keep me going. I pray that this book brings you a bounty of souls who are ready to be transformed by the love of God, just as you were on that mountaintop some time ago. Thank you specifically to Jill Dailey Smith—and you know why.

The Revelation Wellness friends and partners: Thank you for embracing our weird. Whether you found us on a podcast or a friend dragged you to a Revelation Fitness class and now you are marvelously ruined, thank you! I believe every calorie you burn and every breathless declaration you speak in front of your TV (or wherever you move with us) is making momentum for this freedom movement of God. Your prayers and support for using fitness as a tool to spread the gospel message are making our God-sized dream come true. Together we will continue to punch physical and spiritual poverty in the teeth! Every tribe, tongue, and nation will know this freedom message because of you. Thank you.

The Tyndale team: I couldn't have asked for a better first-time publishing experience. I thank God that He chose you for me for such a time as this. Thank you for believing in this wellness mission, which goes far beyond telling people what to eat or how to move. Thank you all for using your time and talent to make this message as excellent as possible. And thank you to Jan Long Harris for getting on a plane, lacing up your sneakers, attending one of my fitness classes, and then taking me to lunch to hear more about my story. Thank you for stepping up to bat for the publishing of this book. Your life-giving words "You are a good writer," spoken to me over a bowl of chips and guacamole, chased away many instances of writer's block.

My editor: Where would the literary world be without editors like you, Kim Miller? You are truly the unsung hero of this book. I pray that Jesus one day shares with you every story of personal transformation and freedom this book creates. You took all my passionate ramblings and put them into proper working order so the world could enjoy a finished work of art—one that comforts and challenges its readers. You're truly the best! Thank you. (And thank you for teaching me the ins and outs of track changes, although I am not sure I ever mastered the skill.)

Moving Forward Journal

Week #: _____ Date: _____

Scripture verse of the week: _____

Meal	Time	Food Eaten	Drink	Hunger Scale Before	Hunger Scale After
Breakfast				1 2 3 4 5 Comments:	1 2 3 4 5
Snack				1 2 3 4 5	1 2 3 4 5
Lunch				1 2 3 4 5 Comments:	1 2 3 4 5
Snack				1 2 3 4 5	1 2 3 4 5
Dinner				1 2 3 4 5 Comments:	1 2 3 4 5
Snack				1 2 3 4 5	1 2 3 4 5
Water	(1) (2) (3) (4) (5) (6) (7) (8) glasses				
Exercise				Prayer/Devotional/Quiet Time Yes No	

Daily Thoughts/Revelation: _____

Wellness Revelation Workout Calendar

An 8-Week Journey

Day 1	Day 2	Day 3	Day 4	Day 5	Day 6	Day 7
Meet Your Trainer	Complete and (If You're in a Group) Turn In Your Action Plan	To Weigh or Not to Weigh	Health Assessment: Stress	Health Assessment: Cardiovascular System	Rest	Rest
Day 8	**Day 9**	**Day 10**	**Day 11**	**Day 12**	**Day 13**	**Day 14**
Health Assessment: Strength	Health Assessment: Endurance	Health Assessment: Flexibility	Rest	Health Assessment: Sleep	Health Assessment: Hydration	Rest
Day 15	**Day 16**	**Day 17**	**Day 18**	**Day 19**	**Day 20**	**Day 21**
Posture and Alignment Training	Healthy Feet and Ankles, Part 1	Healthy Feet and Ankles, Part 2	Healthy Knees	Rest	Stability Training	Rest
Day 22	**Day 23**	**Day 24**	**Day 25**	**Day 26**	**Day 27**	**Day 28**
Mobility Workout	Cardio Dance and Drums Workout	Basic Strength Workout	Rest	Mobility Workout	Podcast Walk	Rest
Day 29	**Day 30**	**Day 31**	**Day 32**	**Day 33**	**Day 34**	**Day 35**
Basic Strength Workout/Stretch	Cardio Dance and Drums Workout	Total Body Strength Workout	Flexibility Training	Rest: "Be Still and Be Loved" Podcast	Cardio and Strength Workout/Stretch	Rest: "Be Still and Be Loved" Podcast

To access each day's assignment, visit revelationwellness.org/book/workout.

Wellness Revelation Workout Calendar
An 8-Week Journey

Day 36	Day 37	Day 38	Day 39	Day 40	Day 41	Day 42
Cardio and Strength Workout/Stretch	Cardio Dance and Drums Workout	Flexibility Training	Podcast Workout	Basic Strength Workout/Stretch	Rest: "Be Still and Be Loved" Podcast	Rest

Day 43	Day 44	Day 45	Day 46	Day 47	Day 48	Day 49
Metabolic Workout (Peak Fitness with Alisa)/Stretch	Yoga Fusion	Podcast Workout	Basic Strength Workout	Hip Release Training	Kickboxing/Stretch	Rest: "Be Still and Be Loved" Podcast

Day 50	Day 51	Day 52	Day 53	Day 54	Day 55	Day 56
Cardio Dance and Drums Workout/Stretch	Basic Strength Workout	Cardio and Strength Workout/Stretch	Kickboxing	Yoga Fusion	Metabolic Workout	Rest

Day 57	Fitness Assessment	Before	After
Reassess Your Health (Redo videos for Days 4–5, 8–10, and 12–13.)	Resting heart rate	_____	_____
	Blood pressure (if known)	_____	_____
	Three-minute step	_____	_____
	Push-ups	_____	_____
	Sit-ups	_____	_____
	Sit and reach	_____	_____
	Hours of sleep	_____	_____
	Ounces of water per day	_____	_____

The LORD has done great things for us, and we are filled with joy.

—Psalm 126:3

To access each day's assignment, visit revelationwellness.org/book/workout.

NOTES

1. Dictionary.com, s.v. "whole."
2. "Obesity and Overweight," National Center for Health Statistics, Centers for Disease Control and Prevention, accessed February 13, 2017, https://www.cdc.gov/nchs/fastats/obesity-overweight.htm.
3. *American Dictionary of the English Language*, s.v. "covenant," http://webstersdictionary1828.com /dictionary/covenant.
4. *English Oxford Living Dictionaries*, s.v. "covenant: theology," https://en.oxforddictionaries.com /definition/covenant.
5. Brennan Manning, in "What If I Stumble?" by Daniel Joseph and Toby McKeehan, *Jesus Freak*, ForeFront/Virgin, 1995.
6. "Obesity and Overweight" National Center for Health Statistics, Centers for Disease Control and Prevention, accessed February 13, 2017, https://www.cdc.gov/nchs/fastats/obesity-overweight.htm.
7. *Merriam-Webster's Collegiate Dictionary*, 11th ed., s.v. "enrich."
8. Latetia V. Moore and Frances E. Thompson, "Adults Meeting Fruit and Vegetable Intake Recommendations—United States, 2013," *Morbidity and Mortality Weekly Report* 64, no. 26 (July 10, 2015): 709–713.
9. Eric Carle, *The Very Hungry Caterpillar* (New York: Philomel Books, 1994), 15.
10. Frederick Buechner, interview by Bob Abernethy, *Religion and Ethics Newsweekly*, PBS, May 5, 2006, http://www.pbs.org/wnet/religionandethics/?p=15358.
11. *Merriam-Webster's Collegiate Dictionary*, 11th ed., s.v. "sufficiency."
12. Bruce Springsteen, "Hungry Heart," *The River*, Columbia Records, 1980.
13. "Resistance Training for Health and Fitness," American College of Sports Medicine, accessed February 13, 2017, https://www.acsm.org/docs/brochures/resistance-training.pdf.
14. *English Oxford Living Dictionaries*, s.v. "transform," https://en.oxforddictionaries.com/definition/us /transform.
15. Deborah S. Hartz-Seeley, "Chronic Stress Is Linked to the Six Leading Causes of Death," *Miami Herald*, March 21, 2014, http://www.miamiherald.com/living/article1961770.html.
16. Oswald Chambers, "The Purpose of Prayer," in *My Utmost for His Highest*, ed. James Reimann (Grand Rapids, MI: Discovery House, 2010), August 28.
17. Robert L. Thomas, ed., *New American Standard Exhaustive Concordance of the Bible with Hebrew-Aramaic and Greek Dictionaries* (Nashville, Holman Bible Publishers, 1981), s.v. "shalom."
18. John MacArthur, *The MacArthur Bible Commentary* (Nashville: Thomas Nelson, 2005), 1621.

ABOUT THE AUTHOR

Alisa Keeton is a wholehearted pursuer of God's love. After more than twenty-five years as a fitness professional, Alisa felt God leading her to bring fresh meaning to the world of health and fitness. At first she resisted, but eventually she got on her knees, rolled up her sleeves, and followed His call. In 2011, she launched Revelation Wellness. This nonprofit ministry uses fitness as a tool to spread the gospel message, inviting participants to become whole and live well. The Revelation Wellness instructor training program equips and sends out "fitness missionaries" throughout the United States and around the world, while RevWell TV brings faith-based online workouts and resources to anyone with Internet access.

Alisa lives in Phoenix with her husband, Simon, and their two children, Jack and Sophia. As a family, they are on mission to change the world with the kind and courageous love of God.

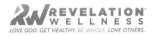

LOVE GOD. GET HEALTHY. BE WHOLE. LOVE OTHERS.

OTHER OFFERINGS OF REVELATION WELLNESS

REVELATION WELLNESS INSTRUCTOR TRAINING
Our nine-week instructor-training course thoroughly equips leaders of all ages, experience levels, and styles to use fitness as a tool to spread the Good News of the gospel message.
www.revelationwellness.org/rwit

LIVE REVELATION FITNESS CLASSES AND WELLNESS REVELATION FACILITATORS
Find a Revelation Fitness class or Wellness Revelation facilitator near you.
www.revelationwellness.org/classes

REVWELL TV
Can't get to a live Revelation Fitness class? Become a monthly partner with Revelation Wellness! Our gift of thanks to you is online access to more than one hundred faith-filled workouts, workshops, wellness resources, and Bible studies.
www.revelationwellness.org/revwell-tv

THE WELLNESS REVELATION AT-HOME STUDY
Want to go deeper in the Wellness Revelation? Join Alisa Keeton in this eight-week self-paced video series designed to help you get to the root of what weighs you down. Let Alisa take you further into the heart of God's love—a love that sets you free and keeps you whole.
www.revelationwellness.org/wellnessrevelation-athome

THE WELLNESS REVELATION ONLINE FACILITATION
Join an online small group led by a highly trained Wellness Revelation facilitator. This eight-week, nine-session course will give you the community and accountability you are looking for.
www.revelationwellness.org/wellnessrevelation-online

REVELATION WELLNESS EVENTS:

RIM TO HIM
Rim to Him is a one-of-a-kind, coed adventure/fund-raiser that culminates in a one-day hike of the Grand Canyon. Our five-month training program is designed to prepare you in heart, mind, soul, and strength to cross one of the wonders of the world! "With God all things are possible" (Matthew 19:26, NIV).
www.revelationwellness.org/events/r2h/

REV ON THE ROAD
Rev on the Road is a two-day outreach and wellness event designed to restore people's hope, faith, and love as image bearers of a good and whole God. Invite Revelation Wellness to come to your city and start a Holy Spirit fire of freedom!
www.revelationwellness.org/events/rotr/

CP1275

Online Discussion *guide*

TAKE *your* TYNDALE READING EXPERIENCE *to the* NEXT LEVEL

A FREE discussion guide for this book
is available at bookclubhub.net, perfect
for sparking conversations in your book
group or for digging deeper into the text
on your own.

www.bookclubhub.net

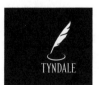

*You'll also find free discussion guides for
other Tyndale books, e-newsletters, e-mail
devotionals, virtual book tours, and more!*